Purple Haze

The Cannabinoid Chronicles Series: Book 1

Written by:
Dawn Peacock

Dedication

This book is dedicated to all those who dream. Don't. Stop. Dreaming. You're the reason the world keeps spinning.

And to all those who love and support dreamers, thank you.

Acknowledgments

Here's where I get to show my love for everyone that helped and supported me. This could be a book in itself, so I'll do my best to keep it concise!

I am beyond grateful for:

Karl and Collin for being such supportive, loving, inspirational and caring sons

Bob Doyle, Sara Barrett, Cheryl Bland, Leanne Rivers, Marie-Pierre Gosselin and Jay Stevenson for lending me their courage when I had none

Sara Barrett, Vicki Wilson Conley, Jane McArthur and Dickey Bill Wagner for your contributions and proofreading

Brittny Arbour for letting me borrow your persona to get the book going

Tina Williams, Vicki Wilson Conley, Marina Carlstein, and Leanne Rivers for your help and guidance in all the stuff AFTER you write the book

Monty Seitz for so, so much - giving me the idea to write this book on CBD as a novel rather than a guide; being an amazing editor and standing your ground when I would throw a fit; believing in me and supporting me in ways that I didn't realize any person could; and helping me to find myself again after having been lost. I am so grateful for having you in my life. I

can truly say that this book would not have been written
without you.

Table of Contents

Chapter 1

"Beatrice, I can't believe you have to leave in a few days. It feels like you just got here a day or two ago."

"I know, Mum, but I start my job a week from Monday and the van will be here anytime to move my things to Colorado. I just need to finish up a few more boxes and then I'm yours until my flight out Friday." Beatrice paused from packing long enough to hug her mom and kiss her on the forehead.

Her mom, Mary, was a petite little thing and British to the core. Her parents had emigrated from the UK when her father accepted an Endowed Professorship at University of Chicago in the 80's. Beatrice was welcomed into the world a few years after. Growing up, she split her time between the UK and the states while attending boarding school in Britain. Bea had just completed her PhD in Biochemistry at Aberdeen University and was happy to be back in the states to start her career.

"I wish your father was still with us to see what you've accomplished. He'd be so proud. He was always so very proud of you, love."

"I know, and I wish he were here as well."

"You were always his 'mini-me' – bright as the sun, stubborn as an ass, and his same odd sense of humor. You'd follow him everywhere like a little parrot. Such a cheeky one! And now you're Dr. Beatrice Clarke! And off to Colorado to study 'pot' of all things. What an amazing world we live in."

"I don't know about the whole "amazing world" bit, but there is a lot of research that needs to be done on cannabis and I'm happy to be a part of it. They've got a real leg up on it here compared to the UK. I'm looking forward to sorting some of this out. CBD doesn't appear to be as promising and safe as all the talk you hear. There are a couple drugs that the FDA has approved here in the states, but that definitely doesn't mean that cannabis is safe for the public. It just means that, under doctor care, there are indications where cannabis is an option for treatment."

"Like my fibromyalgia . . . " Mary interjected.

"Mum, we've been over this. The science is still out on cannabis and fibromyalgia. It's just anecdotal evidence. There are no studies proving that it benefits fibro, or that it's even safe."

"My Facebook Fibro group swears by CBD! Every day I hear someone else talking about how it's helping them. I really think I should try it. They say that you can't get high with CBD - that it's not cannabis, it's hemp."

"Mum, you're not trying it until I know it's safe. We've been over this. I know that you're suffering but for all we know, cannabis could make it worse. Just give me some time. Hemp and cannabis are scientifically the same genus and species – cannabis sativa. CBD is one of the cannabinoids found in the plant that is NOT intoxicating - while THC is another cannabinoid that IS intoxicating. Don't worry. We'll get it sorted. Dr. Sarcos is a brilliant researcher, and although he was a real pain to work under at Aberdeen, I'm really looking forward to working with him on this. Who knows? Maybe we'll be able to participate in some drug trials and get something fast tracked that can help you."

"I can't wait forever, Beatrice. I think it's worth trying, even if it might make it worse. I'm just so tired and the medication isn't working. Can't I just try it?"

"Please. For me. Just give me a couple months to get things going at the job and I promise you that it'll be one of the first things that I focus on. I promise."

Beatrice wrapped her arms around her mother and held her. She wished she could take the pain away. She wished she could help her sleep and give her the energy she used to have, but CBD wasn't a magic-bullet and giving her something that might make things worse just wasn't an option.

"Mum, how about you go take a rest while I finish up here and afterwards I'll take you down to Lake Shore for a cup of tea and we can sit and watch the sunset like Dad used to do."

"I'd like that, dear. I'll just rest up a bit."

"I love you, Mum."

"I love you, too, Beatrice. I love you, too."

Mary made her way to her room and gingerly positioned herself on her bed, tucking pillows here and there to relieve some of the pain and pressure that plagued her body. It had been years since she'd gotten a full night of sleep, always being woken by muscle pain and tingling and burning in her hands and arms. But she trusted her daughter and would wait – impatiently – for Beatrice to give her the okay to join the others in the group that were taking CBD and seemingly doing so well with it. She just hoped that it would be sooner rather than later.

"OK, Izzie," Bea cooed to her pup. "Mummie's got to go to her first day of work. You be a good girl while I'm gone!"

Bea kissed her cock-a-poo on the top of her head and placed her on her pink princess pillow on the couch. That was Miss Izzie's throne and, while it did not match anything in the well-decorated living room of ecru and light blue, it had a prominent place and definitely was indicative of her status in the household. This was Izzie's world and everyone was just playing their part in it.

Bea pulled her Camry out of the 2-car garage at the house she was renting in Fort Collins. It was a nice house, nothing overly special about it, but at two grand a month she was glad to have a six-figure salary to pay for it. Northern Colorado was beautiful and a lot less crowded than Denver, but it was growing fast and living in a college town didn't help the rents any.

It was early June and the clear blue Colorado sky wasn't disappointing. She caught a glimpse of the orange sunrise earlier from her bedroom window when she woke up, but it faded long before she hit the road for work. It was definitely sunglasses time as she drove east into work with the sun trying its best to see how small it could make Bea's pupils. Fortunately, it was a short drive to the office.

The lab, though small, was well equipped. It made the university's lab look shabby by comparison. There was nothing lacking and it was obvious that no expense was spared. From the supercritical CO2 extractor, to the chemistry analyzer, to the mass spectrometer, the lab was as high tech and stocked as it could be. There was no question that there was big money behind this project. Even the lab chairs were top of the line.

As Bea made her way down the hallway, Dr. William Sarcos appeared from his office and greeted her.

"Your office is across from mine," Bill Sarcos said curtly. "Go ahead and drop your things in there and meet me in my office. Bring a notepad."

He disappeared back into his office.

Bea entered her office and was quite pleased. She didn't have a window, but it was spacious and bright and even had a meeting table and a couch. Her desk faced the door so she could see who was walking by, and although it didn't look directly into Dr. Sarcos' office, if she moved her chair a bit, she could see into it. The hallway floors were tile – typical for a lab - but both offices had plush carpeting with a padding that made it feel like you were walking on air. She figured she could sleep on that carpet if need be – forget about the couch! From the solid light-oak desk to the mini-fridge to the plush carpet – nothing but the best.

Bea grabbed a notepad and a pen from her desk and went into Dr. Sarcos' office. He was finishing up a call and waved her towards a seat opposite him at his desk.

"No, bring in the oil from China," Sarcos demanded over the phone. "We're using that for this run. We get the results we need that way. I need it by Friday."

Sarcos hung up the phone and turned to Bea, "Let's get to it. We already know each other from the labs in Aberdeen so we don't need to go through any of the niceties. The HR company said you've filled out all of your paperwork and passed the background and drug tests so all that's behind us. If you have any questions about that stuff, call them. I don't involve myself in any of that. You're going to be working mostly with me. The Lab Rats will be doing the dirty work. You'll be analyzing the results under my direction and will be fine-tuning my notes and reviewing communications before they go out. Do you have any questions about the NDA you signed?"

"No."

"Good. Because we enforce that. We spend as much money on lawyers as we do on lab equipment and you can see how much money we spend on that."

"Yes, understood."

"How much experience do you have with cannabinoids?"

"None really."

"I'm glad. It's hard to find people that don't already have it stuck in their minds that they're the cure-all for everything. They're not. And we're going to prove that. We're very well-funded to be able to prove that. We have all of the tools at our disposal to be able to show that cannabinoids are dangerous and need to be scheduled by the FDA as such. They need to remain under the control of the FDA, and only be available through the pharmaceutical industry. Understood?"

"Yes, okay. Like I said, I don't have any experience in that area and its obviously your area of expertise, so I look forward to learning from you."

"Fine," Sarcos turned to his computer. "I'm emailing you a list of standard terms that you'll need to familiarize yourself with. I'm also sending you two white papers that I've recently published. Review these as they will be the basis of what we're building on here. We have a meeting Wednesday with a pharma rep that we're working with. I want you to sit in and listen. I also have a set of lab results that I need you to log. You can look at the prior ones that I've done and figure it out from there. If you have any questions, let me know."

"Thank you. I'll get right on it."

Bea got out of her chair and by the time she reached the door he was on the phone again.

"Well, at least that answers that question," she thought to herself. "He's still an ass."

Bea spent the day getting settled and dove into the list of terms and white papers that Dr. Sarcos had sent her. Some of the terminology was familiar to her from her chemistry and botany studies, but there were others that were very cannabis-specific.

Cannabinoid: chemical compounds that act on cannabinoid receptors in cells that alter a neurotransmitter release in the brain

Cannabidiol: also known as CBD - a nonintoxicating phytocannabinoid isolated in 1940 in cannabis and hemp; second most prevalent cannabinoid found in most cannabis plants behind THC

Tetrahydrocannabinol: also known as THC - the principal psychoactive constituent of cannabis; a lipid found in cannabis; first isolated in 1964

Endocannabinoid: any of several chemical compounds (such as anandamide) that are naturally produced within the body (human or animal) and bind to the same brain receptors as compounds derived from cannabis

<u>Phytocannabinoid</u>: cannabinoids that occur naturally in the cannabis plant

<u>Endocannabinoid/Phytocannabinoid equivalents:</u>
There are equivalents between cannabinoids created within the body (endocannabinoids) and cannabinoids found in the cannabis plant (phytocannabinoids). The major equivalents reported by David A. Dawkins are:
- Anandamide (AEA) & THC
- 2-AG & CBD
- Virodhamine & THCV
- NADA & CBC
- Lysophatidylinsitol & CBG
- Olemide & CBN

"Our bodies make cannabinoids that are biologically equivalent to those found in cannabis?" she asked aloud to nobody in particular. She continued reading, more intrigued than before.

<u>Endocannabinoid System:</u> a biological system composed of endocannabinoids - endogenous lipid-based retrograde neurotransmitters that bind to cannabinoid receptors - and cannabinoid receptor proteins that are expressed throughout the vertebrate central nervous system (including the brain) and peripheral nervous system. In simpler terms, it is a cell-signaling system in the body (human/animal) which plays a role in regulating a range of functions.

Bea started to understand the biochemical synergetic interaction between cannabinoids and the body. If these observations were true, then there could be something to the anecdotes after all.

While doing some additional research online, she ran across the CannabisClinicians.org site, which had a number of resources including research white papers for clinicians organized by numerous conditions.

Included in the research were cannabis white papers on:

- Pain management and mitigation
- Inflammation
- Nervous System Diseases
- Seizures
- Alzheimer's Disease
- Cancer
- Immune System Diseases
- Autism
- Bone Diseases
- Cardiovascular Disease
- Dementia
- Diabetes
- Joint Diseases
- Muscular Diseases
- Addiction
- ADD

Bea was surprised by the amount of information that was available, as she was under the impression that everything was simply anecdotal. But just because there were studies and papers, didn't mean it was safe or beneficial.

Chapter 2

Bea's first week at her new job was a hectic one, but nothing that she couldn't handle. Dr. Sarcos was called to Virginia on business, so Wednesday's meeting was cancelled. The majority of her time was spent either playing email ping-pong with him or wading through a barrage of messages that he had forwarded for her to handle. Fortunately, the oil from China had come in a day early, as international shipments weren't on Bea's l-ong list of things she had experience in.

Bea met the "Lab Rats" – most of whom were recent undergrads from CSU – early in the week. Dr. Sarcos had hired these 22 and 23 year-olds straight out of school but had never spent the time with them to train them properly. She was able to offer some pointers that she had learned in grad school to help make their processes easier and they were like puppies gobbling down treats, eating up all the knowledge she could dish out. She noted that she would be able to make measurable advances in the company with minimal effort in that area and was grateful that the "puppies" were so open to learning and advancing their skills.

The most important connection that Bea made in her first week was with Sheila, Dr. Sarcos' personal assistant. Sheila was a tiny woman – barely over 5 feet even in heels - in her late 50's to early 60's, and very soft spoken. While the rest of the office was attired in office casual, you would never find Sheila in anything less than a dress, hose and heels and a full face of makeup. Her desk was always impeccably clean without even a paperclip out of place. She was a throw-back to an earlier time in the business world, where roles were clearly demarcated and secretaries, rather than personal assistants, truly did manage their bosses' lives both inside and outside of the office. Sheila did everything from paying Dr. Sarcos' personal bills, scheduling his laundry pickup, car maintenance, house cleaning, grocery delivery and medical appointments to also managing his calendar, flights, expense reports and more. A single woman who never married or had children, Sheila started working for Dr. Sarcos 20 years prior when he was project manager for a research project in a lab back east. He hasn't scheduled a haircut, ordered a meal or even bought underwear on his own since.

By the end of the week, Bea had her schedule down and felt competent in her daily tasks and was ready to take on bigger ones. Even Miss Izzie had settled into a routine at home which made Bea's life that much easier.

It was Saturday afternoon, and earlier in the day Bea had ticked another item off her to-do list: finding the perfect place for her monthly mani-pedi. While Dr. Sarcos may not tout the benefits of a work-life balance, she knew that a killer pedicure could change the course of history – especially with the right polish choice. Invigorated by her monthly indulgence, she grabbed a water bottle, collapsible bowl and Izzie and made her way to Horsetooth Reservoir for a little exercise. The weather was perfect and she was antsy to experience some of the hiking trails in the area. Izzie – not so much.

Horsetooth Reservoir was located west of the city near CSU's old football stadium and was named after a large rock formation in the area that resembled a large tooth from – you guessed it - a horse. It covered 1,900 acres and was filled with snow runoff from the mountains. As it was already midday, the reservoir was filled with watercraft of different shapes and sizes, and hikers of all ages peppered the trails in the park – several with dogs in tow.

Bea put Izzie down at the base of a rock at the top of the trail where she stopped for a breather. Izzie had made it an entire five minutes before planting herself firmly in the middle of the trail, refusing to budge. No coaxing was going to convince Izzie to use her legs, so Bea scooped her up and carried her to the top of the trail where the view was just as she had seen on numerous Instagram posts. She added her own version to the plethora of #horsetooth contributions but this one featured Izzie with her "over it" expression which would no doubt garner a hundred hearts or so.

While trying to convince Izzie that the downhill walk would be much easier than the uphill trek, Bea suddenly heard the sound of branches breaking, some rather descriptive expletives and a dog barking loudly in the distance.

"Damn rookies," she heard as she headed in the direction of the commotion to see if she could somehow be of assistance. "Share the fucking trails!"

As Bea reached the junction of the trail, she saw a yellow lab standing above the drop-off, wagging his tail furiously while holding a stick in his mouth. Following the dog's line of sight, she could see the figure of a man making his way up the hill through the trees and brush.

"It's not funny, Rufus," he yelled up at the yellow lab. But Rufus' "full-body butt wiggle" showed he disagreed.

"Hey, do you need a hand?" Bea yelled down to the figure coming closer into view. And oh, what a view. "You got wrecked!" she exclaimed, seeing the shirtless man come into a clearing – scraped and slightly bloodied from his tumble down the hill. What a shame, as that torso was about as close to perfect as she'd ever seen.

"No, I'm good. Just a couple clueless kids on bikes that were in way over their heads to be on this trail. Way too technical for them." He reached up and grabbed the trunk of a small tree to pull himself up the last bit of the incline and onto level ground. Rufus started jumping around gleefully – stick still firmly held between the canine's canines – while Izzie looked on from the safety of her mother's arms with hesitation.

"Jaime," he said, extending his hand in greeting.

"Beatrice, but you can call me Bea," she said, shifting Izzie to her left arm to meet his hand half-way with her right.

He shook her hand and she noticed that his hands were soft and he had a firm – but not aggressively so – handshake. She looked up to see the most amazing hazel eyes – speckled green and brown that looked like a mosaic - and immediately looked down at her feet as she became self-conscious from staring for too long.

"Can I offer you some water to clean you up?" she quickly asked, putting Izzie down and taking her backpack off to retrieve the water and a bandana. "It's no trouble. Really."

"Uh, sure." Jaime checked himself and took inventory of his cuts and soon-to-be bruises. The drop-off had quite a few rocks and the worst of his injuries was a gash on his back. He tried to look over his left shoulder to assess it.

"Here, let me take a look," Bea offered.

Jaime turned around to let her see. "Oh, that's gonna leave a scar." She poured water on the wound and cleaned up the blood that trickled down his back into his shorts. "Focus, Bea," she told herself as she moved her wet bandana over his broad back soaking up the glistening water that she had poured on him to rinse off the blood. "It doesn't look like it needs stitches, but it's definitely going to leave a scar."

"No worries. I'll just put a little CBD on it and it'll heal up."

"Well, at least he's pretty," Bea thought to herself, noting that he'd been drinking the CBD Kool-Aid.

"Neomycin might be a better choice," she offered. "You might not want to risk getting an infection with this."

"CBD's an anti-bacterial. It'll work fine and it'll also work on any inflammation so it won't scar as badly. I'm good."

"Oh, OK," she replied, wondering if it really was an anti-bacterial as she hadn't seen anything about that in Dr. Sarcos' white papers. But she wasn't about to bring that up now as she was enjoying her chance encounter with Mr. Outdoorsy McBody.

Jaime turned around and Bea started washing the scrapes on his chest without thinking. Realizing what she was doing, she jumped back in embarrassment and tripped backwards over Izzie, landing smack on her butt.

"Oh my gosh, I'm so sorry! I shouldn't have . . . I wasn't thinking," she stammered.

"Quite all right. I wasn't going to stop you. Let me help you up." He reached out and took Bea's hand while wrapping his other arm around her back to bring her upright. Rufus had abandoned his stick at this point and was sniffing Izzie curiously, which she was tolerating - for now.

Bea brushed the dirt off her shorts and shirt. "Need any help?" Jaime offered.

"No, I'll be quite fine," she giggled shyly.

"How about a beer at Odell's? It's getting warm and personally, I've had enough adventure for one day."

"Odell's? What about the dogs?"

"You're new to Fort Collins, aren't you?"

"How'd you know?"

"One: everyone around here knows that Odell's is dog friendly. Two: you've got a *lovely accent*," he offered, using his best British accent imitation, "And, three: I would have noticed you if you'd been here for more than a few months. You're stunning."

Bea turned all shades of red and pink and stuttered and stammered through an embarrassing acceptance of his offer as they made their way down the trail to the parking lot. Even Izzie was happy to traverse the worn dirt trail down to the trailhead with an occasional nose in the butt from Rufus who had long lost interest in his stick and was now more interested in his new friend.

Odell Brewing was humming, but there were a few empty tables on the patio where the dogs were welcome. A slight breeze made its way from the foothills, providing relief from the hot sun. Jaime – now fully clothed to Bea's dismay – grabbed a flight of beers for Bea to taste and a pint of Myrecenary – a double IPA – for himself. The dogs relaxed in the shade of the table and napped while the humans got to know each other better.

"So how long have you been here?"

"Just a couple weeks. My new job started Monday."

"Where are you working?"

"Medicroy Labs near the HP campus. I'm the senior project analyst overseeing research and development. What about you?"

"I'm a vet – companion animals. I'm participating in a research project with CSU. I've done a lot of work with them since I graduated a few years back. As an alum, they call me in whenever something good comes up. What are you researching?"

"Actually, I'm not allowed to discuss it. Their NDA is pretty tight and they're lawyered up. I'd probably have to kill you if I told you."

"I could think of worse ways to die."

Chapter 3

The glow from Bea's weekend outing had faded within minutes of being at the office. With Dr. Sarcos back, Monday felt like a mental marathon. He downloaded a week's worth of information to organize and disseminate, in addition to setting out an agenda for the next few days that was Herculean at best. The Lab Rats were scurrying to finish their final testing on the oil from China, Sheila was making quick work of going through a stack of receipts and notes to transcribe from Dr. Sarcos, and the man, himself, was holed up in his office making call after call.

It was nearly noon before Bea came up for air. She had filled her mini fridge with fruit, cheese and her favorite bubbly water for lunches for the week, knowing that the first few days with Dr. Sarcos would probably be overwhelming. She grabbed some snacks and ate at her desk while wading through data and charting results. Dr. Sarcos had brought back data from a study he was overseeing in Virginia and was getting ready to start a new one with the oil from China. The Virginia study was conducted using Colorado oil and, while Dr. Sarcos was adamant that CBD had no beneficial effects, the data from the double-blind study that Bea was charting suggested just the opposite.

"Bea, when you get a chance?" Dr. Sarcos called from his office.

"On my way," Bea answered back as she rolled her chair back

and started towards his door.

"Close the door," he instructed.

Bea closed the door behind her and walked towards his desk.

"How's the charting coming along?"

"It's coming along well. I've gotten all but the last subset entered. I should have it all in by the end of the hour."

"Good, we'll be duplicating that study with the Chinese oil so keep the data handy. We're going to be comparing the results weekly. The Chinese oil will give us the data that we need over the Colorado oil, but we may be able to find some data to pull from the local oil as well."

"Yeah, I was a little surprised at what I was seeing from the Virginia study. I didn't expect to see results like that."

"Data can be deceiving. The oil from China will give us what we need. I doubt I'll be using any of the results from the Virginia participants – just the next set. Chart them and we'll have it archived to use as a comparison, and if I can find anything of use from it, I'll pull it out."

"Will do."

"And remember, this data falls under your NDA, so no information about this leaves your office – not even to the Lab Rats."

"Got it."

"Get with Sheila about ordering in for dinner. We're going to have a late night tonight."

Bea sat at her desk eating the food brought in from Honolulu Poke – a poke bowl with brown rice, octopus, scallop and salmon with a Yuzu Citrus sauce – reviewing more of the notes and white papers that Dr. Sarcos had given her to get her up to speed on CBD and the endocannabinoid system.

<u>Cannabinoid Receptor:</u> located throughout the body, part of the endocannabinoid system; are of a class of cell membrane receptors in the G protein-coupled receptor superfamily.

<u>Terpene:</u> any of a large group of volatile unsaturated hydrocarbons found in the essential oils of plants

<u>Endocannabinoid Deficiency:</u> also known as CED (Clinical Endocannabinoid Deficiency). Dr. Ethan Russo published multiple papers on the topic, "If endocannabinoid function were decreased, it follows that a lowered pain threshold would be operative, along with derangements of digestion, mood, and sleep among the almost universal physiological systems subserved by the endocannabinoid system (ECS)."

She turned to Dr. Russo's 2016 paper, *Clinical Endocannabinoid Deficiency Reconsidered*, and started making notes in one of her notebooks that she kept in her oversized purse. Specifically, she looked for references that could support or contradict the efficacy of CBD for treating fibromyalgia to look into later for her mother.

Bea moved on to one of Dr. Sarcos' white papers that discussed the marketing and sales of CBD.

<u>CBD marketing terms:</u>
- Full spectrum – product containing full plant cannabinoids including some amount of THC
- Broad spectrum – product containing full plant cannabinoids with the exception of THC
- Isolate – isolated CBD molecule
- Distillate - a highly refined cannabis extract often derived from high CBD hemp flower and hemp biomass. CBD Distillate typically contains around 80% CBD with the balance including minor cannabinoids, terpenes and other plants oils and extracts.

The remaining white papers contained much more information citing other papers and PubMed articles listed by the National Institute of Health.

She went back to her charting with a new respect for the potential of cannabinoids in treating certain conditions, but more confused as to why Dr. Sarcos' position was so contrary to the use of them. Especially when the results from the study were showing just the opposite of what he was saying.

By the time Bea got home, Izzie's four legs were crossed to the point she could barely hold her need to pee before she got outside. She was NOT amused that her human didn't get home until well after 9pm and let her know in no uncertain terms. If looks could kill, Bea would be six feet under.

"I'm so sorry! I couldn't leave," Bea explained to Izzie. "Dr. Sarcos had to have the results charted and the new oil prepared for the next round. I didn't have a choice. But I saved some of my dinner for you."

Bea set the contents of the doggie bag from the Honolulu Poke Bar in Izzie's bowl, hoping to break the wall of ice that she had put up. Fortunately, Izzie needed to eat as badly as she had needed to pee moments before, so all was forgiven.

It was nearly 10pm before Bea grabbed her phone to jump online to see what the rest of the world was doing. First up was Instagram to look at an array of pics from cute puppies to selfies of friends to Instant Pot recipes. Next was a quick glance at Reddit and then on to Snapchat – where a snap was waiting patiently to be opened.

She didn't recognize the name at first, but when she opened the picture, her heart skipped a beat. Dr. Hotty McVet had snapped a pic of himself and Rufus at the reservoir as the sun was setting. It was a great pic but Bea would have preferred a shirtless one to refresh her memory from the hike on Saturday. She resisted the urge to reply to the snap and plugged the phone in to charge for the night.

"Bedtime, Izzie! Where'd you go?" she asked aloud, looking for her pup.

It was odd – Izzie was never more than a few feet away from Bea in the evenings. Bea went room to room looking for Izzie, getting a little more nervous with every blank floor and piece of furniture that she saw. Finally, she walked into the kitchen where she heard a noise. There she found Izzie on the floor, seizing.

Bea immediately threw herself next to Izzie on the floor, calling out to her. "Izzie, Izzie. It's OK. I'm here. It's OK. It's OK." Bea wasn't sure if she was saying that for Izzie's benefit or her own. She sat with her waiting for the seizure to stop, then scooped her up in her arms and rushed to the animal hospital.

Bea filled out the paperwork for Izzie and gave them the info of her previous vet. She sat in the mostly empty waiting room, holding Izzie in her arms and talking quietly to her.

"Izzie?" a kind voice called out, waiting to lead the patient and her human back to the exam room. "Hi, I'm Lisa and I'm going to get some information and vitals on Izzie for the doctor. Can you tell me what happened?"

Bea filled Lisa in on her evening and how she had been really late in getting home and the doggie bag that she had fed Izzie and was feeling like a horrible fur-baby mom. Lisa examined

Izzie and eased Bea's mind that she was sure that there was nothing that Bea had done that evening to trigger the seizure. She left Bea and Izzie in the exam room and told her that a doctor would be with them shortly.

Within a minute or so, an older woman knocked and came into the exam room, introducing herself as Dr. Britton. She was a kind, older woman, probably in her mid-70's, with a soothing voice and a warm disposition – which was immediately overrun when Rufus bounded in, hell bent on getting to Izzie to see what was happening.

"Rufus, NO!" Dr. Britton exclaimed. "I'm so sorry!"

"Rufus, what are you doing here?" Bea asked. Izzie didn't seem to mind as Rufus raised his nose to the examining table, sniffing her to make sure that he was satisfied with the level of care she was receiving.

"Bea?" Jaime asked as he walked into the room, trying to see what the chaos was about. "Is Izzie OK?"

Without warning, tears came pouring from Bea's eyes and she was in a full-blown meltdown. "I had to work late. I didn't get home until after 9. She'd been alone all day and then I gave her leftovers from the Poke Bar and when I went to look for her, she was having a seizure," Bea managed to get out between sobs.

Jaime walked over to Bea and held her in his arms, stroking her hair. Dr. Britton had joined Izzie and Rufus and was examining

Izzie, making notes in her chart.

"How does she look, Mom?" Jaime asked. Bea looked from Jaime to Dr. Britton, assessing this piece of information.

"She looks pretty good, a little weak, but good," she replied. "Was this her first seizure that you know of?"

"Yes, I've never seen her have a seizure before."

"About how long did it last?"

"I'm not sure how long she had been seizing. I was looking for her and calling for her for probably a good minute before I found her and it lasted maybe another 30 seconds after that. She's usually right by my side after work – I just thought she was mad at me."

"It could be an isolated event, but I'd like to keep her for observation."

Bea broke down in tears again as Jaime wrapped his arms around her once more, calming her down. "Rufus and I will keep an eye on her," Jaime assured her. "And I'll call you if anything happens. Why don't you head home and get some rest?"

Bea looked at him, still confused from everything that had just transpired and nodded her head slowly. "OK," she murmured and kissed Izzie on her head, stroking her fur and looking into her big round eyes.

"You be a good girl for Jaime and Dr. Britton. Mommy will come get you tomorrow. I love you," Bea explained to Izzie, holding back tears.

"I'll be right back," Jaime told his mother as he gently took Bea by the arm and walked her out of the exam room and towards her car.

"Are you OK?" he asked Bea as they reached her car.

"No. I have so many questions right now – about Izzie, about you, about why you and Rufus are here . . . "

"We'll talk tomorrow. Just go home and get some rest. My mom and I will take good care of Izzie. She's in excellent hands."

He kissed her on her forehead and opened her car door for her. Bea reluctantly got in and drove away. "By far, the weirdest night of my life," she said to herself. "By far."

Chapter 4

Bea woke up to her cell phone ringing – a number she didn't recognize but, in her morning haze, she answered it anyway.

"Bea, Sarcos here. I need you on a plane to Virginia at 10am. Sheila has booked you a flight and a hotel room. You'll fly back tomorrow. I'm taking the jet and will pick you up at the airport when you land. We have a meeting with a congressman and someone from Gelinex Pharmaceuticals. Dress appropriately. Get with Sheila for the details."

Click.

Bea stared into space, not sure if she had been dreaming or if someone had actually just had the nerve to call her at 5am and hijack the next 24 plus hours of her life. She glanced at her phone and the call log confirmed the latter.

"FUCK!" she yelled to nobody in particular as she got out of bed to let Izzie out. "DOUBLE FUCK!" she exclaimed, remembering the events of last night. Her heart started aching as she remembered seeing Izzie seizing on the kitchen floor and quickly called Jaime to find out how Izzie was doing.

"Uh, hello?" a sleepy voice answered the before dawn call.

"Oh my gosh! I'm so sorry!" Bea whispered. "It's Bea. I forgot the time! I'm so sorry!"

"No worries, it's okay." Jaime stretched, trying to get the blood in his body to start moving. In the background, Bea could hear what sounded like Rufus yawning and possibly some licking.

"It sounds like you've got some company over there. Was that Rufus yawning?"

"Yes, and I didn't realize that Izzie was a morning licker."

"You have Izzie with you? Is she okay?"

"Yeah, she's doing fine. I brought her home with me so I could keep an eye on her. I put a monitor on her and she did have a couple very small seizures during the night. You probably wouldn't have even noticed that she had them if she wasn't on a monitor."

"Oh, no! My poor Izzie!"

"Izzie will be okay. Don't worry. We'll find out what's happening, but now that we know it's not an isolated incident we need to start treating her. Can you stop by the clinic today?"

"Oh, crap! I just got a call from my boss and have to be on a plane at 10am. He woke me from a sound sleep, told me to get on a plane, said I'll be back tomorrow and hung up. I'll call him back and tell him I can't go."

"No, no – you don't need to do that. I'll keep Izzie an extra day. I want to monitor her anyway and see how the oil is working. We may have to adjust it."

"Oil?"

"Yeah, I was going to go over treatment options with you at the clinic, but for seizures we typically start with 5mg CBD oil and titrate up from there until the seizures are controlled."

"What? Isn't there a prescription for seizures that she can take?"

"Yes, but the side effects can be worse than the seizures themselves. We've treated hundreds of dogs with CBD for seizures. I'd say 85% of them don't need anything other than the oil. Do some research, but I can tell you from experience that CBD is safer and more effective than most of the pharmaceuticals out there for seizures in dogs – especially small dogs like Izzie."

"You're serious."

"Very. CBD has a very solid history for treating seizures. Epidiolex is a CBD based FDA approved drug specifically for seizures – and it's just a CBD isolate. Izzie's getting a broad spectrum CBD oil that also contains minor cannabinoids and terpenes – a much better treatment than an isolate. Families are literally moving to states where they can get safe access to CBD because it's saving their children's lives. This isn't snake oil."

"OK, ummmm. I don't really know what to say."

"Bea, I've treated a lot of dogs with seizures. I wouldn't lead you astray on this. I want Izzie to be healthy and I feel this is the best treatment for her. It's definitely the safest."

"You go ahead to Virginia," Jaime continued. "I'll keep Izzie with me and get her on CBD. Let me know when you get back tomorrow night and we'll get together and get Izzie back to you. Although Rufus may not be too happy about that."

"You're sure about this? About keeping Izzie, about the CBD, about the seizures? You're sure about all of this?"

"Yes, everything is going to be OK. I know this has to be very overwhelming for you, but everything is going to be fine."

"I seriously don't know what to say. Thank you."

"Oh, you haven't seen my bill yet! You may want to hold off on that!"

"Of course! I'm happy to pay whatever! I totally expect to see commas in my bill!"

"Actually, I was thinking about dinner at The Rare - we'll talk about that when you get back tomorrow night. But right now, Rufus and Izzie are at the door wanting to go outside, so how about you give me a call tonight if you have time and I'll update you on how she's doing?"

"Jaime, I seriously cannot thank you enough for what you're

doing for me. I don't know what I would have done if I hadn't met you."

"Well, you don't have to worry about that because you DID meet me. But right now Rufus is trying to eat the door, so I have to get going. Have a good flight."

"Thank you! Thank you, so much!"

Bea sat on the edge of her bed and looked around her empty room. Then she realized that she had to leave for the airport in less than two hours and didn't have any clean clothes to pack.

"FUCK!"

Bea arrived at the airport in Virginia and made her way to the pick-up area. Dr. Sarcos had emailed her to let her know where the driver would meet her. He had gone straight to the meeting and instructed her to meet him there. The driver was theirs for the duration of their stay, so she could leave her luggage with him.

As she got closer to the designated area, she saw dozens of drivers holding whiteboards with names scrawled on them - names written in English, French, Farsi and Arabic; company names; names of countries and departments of government; and a handful of kids holding hand-made posters with family members' names. What she didn't see was anything with her name on it.

Bea pulled out her phone and read the email again, checking the time to see if maybe she was early or late. No, she was on time and she was exactly where the email instructed her to be. Dr. Sarcos was already at the meeting, waiting for her, so calling him was not an option. She did the next best thing – she called Sheila.

"Dr. Sarcos' office, " Sheila answered. "How may I help you?"

"Hi Sheila, it's Bea. I'm at the airport and I'm having trouble finding my ride."

"He should be there. I set it up myself and he texted me not ten minutes ago to say he was there."

"I'm where Dr. Sarcos' email instructed me to go, but I don't see my name or the lab name on any of the signs."

"Oh, you won't see our name on there. Look for Gelinex Pharmaceuticals. It will be under their name."

"Oh, OK," Bea looked around. Sure enough, there was a tall man in a black suit holding a neatly printed poster with "Gelinex Pharmaceuticals" printed in big bold letters, along with a logo. "Found him," she told Sheila and thanked her for her help.

Ed was an elderly man, 6'2" or so, with a dark tan, a crop of white hair on his head, and a gold chain around his neck. He looked a bit out of place standing next to the other drivers who looked more "corporate" with their starched collars and neatly cut hair, standing at attention waiting for their riders. Ed was leaning up against a pillar, scrolling through his phone with one hand, holding the poster askew with the other.

"Hi, I'm Bea," she said as she approached Ed.

"OK," he mumbled and turned and walked towards the car. "This way."

Ed hadn't uttered a word on the walk to the car, but instead was intently looking at his phone. When they got to the black Escalade, he went directly to the driver's door, got in and started the car. Bea let herself in the back door, pushing her suitcase in before her. As she closed the door she surveyed the Escalade – black leather interior, Elvis on the radio, and a small medallion of what looked to be a saint hanging from the rear view mirror. What had she gotten herself into?

Chapter 5

Ed pulled up to a small, non-descript building in an industrial part of town. There was no sign, other than a marker with the address, to indicate what the business was that occupied the building.

"That's you," he said impatiently, waiting for Bea to get out of the car. "You can leave your stuff here. I'll pick you and Bill up later."

"Bill?" Bea asked.

"Yeah, Bill Sarcos. You're with Billy, right?"

"Oh, yes. Sorry. Of course. Jet lag brain," Bea let herself out of the car. "Thank you."

Bea walked slowly towards the plain, one-story warehouse-like building and surveyed her surroundings. She instinctively put up her guard, noting how these buildings and her driver, Ed, were very familiar and very indicative of places and people that her mom had told her to stay away from. People that made their livings – very good livings – in ways that were an arms-length away from the law. Bea walked slowly to the entrance, both knowing and not knowing what to expect from this meeting with the congressman and pharmaceutical executive. Her level of respect for "Billy" was now as questionable as her surroundings.

Bea took a deep breath, gathered herself, squared her shoulders and hit the button on the door to announce herself. She looked straight into the camera hidden in the corner of the entry and waited for them to answer.

"Name?" said the monotone male voice in the void.

"Dr. Beatrice Clarke," she replied, matching the tone of the hidden requestor.

She heard the familiar buzz of the door lock being deactivated and pushed her way through. The front office was very plain – old, drab carpeting with a handful of non-matching office chairs, a wooden desk with nothing atop it and a large man sitting behind it. What was not so "plain" was the shoulder-strap holster with the revolver in it that the large man was sporting. He smiled, stood up, walked towards the door behind him, punched in a code and opened it for Bea.

"The conference room is the first door on the right. They're waiting for you there. They've been laughing and catching up this morning, so they're in a good mood. You can let your guard down a bit," the guard offered, chuckling.

Bea loosened her shoulders a bit, not realizing that it was so apparent that she was leery of her surroundings. She walked past the "receptionist" and into the hallway towards the conference room. Large voices and bolts of laughter came from the room where even larger men were waiting inside, laughing and slapping each other on the back as she entered. Dr. Sarcos – "Billy" – was the smallest among them, along with two other gentlemen in smart, conservative suits.

Dr. Sarcos regained his composure as he motioned for everyone to take their seats. "Bea, glad you could join us. Take a seat." He pointed to a chair opposite him and between the two conservatively-dressed gentlemen. "This is Dr. Zabini from Gelinex Pharmaceuticals and Representative Jeffries from New Jersey. Gentlemen, this is Bea, my senior project analyst in Colorado."

The two gentlemen stood up and shook Bea's hand while the other men in the room simply sat and stared, saying nothing. Bea sat at the table and readied herself, still not sure what to expect.

"Joey," Dr. Sarcos said, speaking to Representative Jeffries, "Bea compiled the data from the Virginia study for the archives. The Chinese oil version started yesterday. That's the one that we'll be using for our testimony to the Ways and Means Committee with the FDA next month."

"Vinnie," Sarcos continued, shifting his focus to Dr. Zabini. "We'll get you the Colorado oil results for your use. You'll want to pay extra attention to the results in blood sugar levels. They're leveling across the board. We're working on narrowing down the cannabinoid and terpene profile to capitalize on that. Bea, what other levels did you see that benefitted in the first study?"

Startled at the flip-flop on the view of cannabinoids by Dr. Sarcos, Bea stammered, "Umm, I did notice a drop in blood pressure in a large section of the participants who's blood pressure was high coming into the study – but not sure if that was due to experiencing lower anxiety or the blood vessels relaxing."

"Good, we'll want to focus on that as well in the next formulation, Vinnie. Get your guys working on that and put that study under the branded company," Sarcos instructed.

"Will do." Vinnie added, "We're going to need more of the Colorado oil if you want us to use the nano processed tincture for that run. I gave the last of it to Joey for his wife's Crohn's."

"That's right. Joey, how's she doing with that oil?"

"She's great," Joey answered, "She's gaining some of her weight back and is able to get out of the house more. She's still a little nervous about being out for more than an hour, but the longer she takes the CBD, the more she's realizing that she's over the worst of it. She actually had lasagna last night with a big glass of red wine and had no problems all."

"That's amazing – I'm looking forward to going out to dinner with her when she's feeling up to it, like old times."

"Vinnie," Sarcos continued. "Let Bea know how much oil you need for the study and she'll get it to you."

Bea worked hard to keep her jaw from dropping to the table and a poker face intact while watching the complete turnaround on the efficacy of CBD on the part of Dr. Sarcos unfold before her eyes.

Sarcos addressed the group, "Okay, let's focus on what we're expecting from the Chinese oil. Primarily, the heavy metals are going to muddy up the blood sugar numbers and will throw immune indicators off, and may even show some red blood cell mutations if we get some cancer-prone participants. Where are we getting this pool of the China 2 study from?"

"They're Jersey folk – mostly homeless," Vinnie explained. "We're giving them $50 a week for their time and free breakfast and dinner during the study when we give them their doses. They have to commit to showing up every morning and late afternoon to take the tincture. We're not letting any of the oil out of the lab so it doesn't show up in anyone else's hands for them to test it."

"Good idea. We don't need a repeat of what happened last time. Fortunately, using a ghost company name covered our trail on that one. Are we going with low dosing to minimize the benefits, or is the Chinese oil dirty enough to give larger doses to take advantage of the heavy metals?"

"It's only 15% crude, so we're able to go with higher doses on this one. We'll be able to say dosing is 25mg, twice a day, but since the oil is only 15%, we'll get what we need to keep the FDA on our side. And we'll have the other studies to show what we need for the pharma side to move forward with the new FDA approvals for the two drugs we're releasing."

"Have you gotten the other group working on confirming the

results of the first Colorado oil study?"

"Yes, they started the duplicate study the day after the results came in. All signs are showing that it's going to confirm what we found in the first. We have a subset in there with Alzheimer's as well, that we're adding another 30 days to as we're hearing from family members that they're seeing marked improvements in behavior. We may be able to spin that off into another product line. Same oil as the rest, but under another line."

"Two, maybe three products from the same study. That's not bad. We'll have to throw in an additional active ingredient or two to differentiate the products so they don't realize that they're basically the same, and we'll need to spawn some new studies. Let's get started on the patents and trademarks ASAP."

"We'll get that started by Friday. We just need to make sure we get FDA approval before presenting to Congress and launch just after. That way we can show that CBD is dangerous, but that a pharmaceutical company is able to make it safe for use with a doctor's prescription."

"Joey, do you need anything else from us right now?" Sarcos asked.

"Just the presentation materials so I can write up some questions for the committee members to ask," replied Jeffries.

"What about you, Vinnie?" Sarcos asked.

"No, I just need the new Chinese oil study results. I have the results from the first round to match them up to. With a dirtier oil, I think I'm going to have exactly what I need to show the dangers of non-pharma CBD products and keep it all in pharmaceutical companies' hands for our investors."

"Perfect. Bea, I want you to spend time with Vinnie's Director of R&D and go over the Chinese oil results from the previous study we did and what's coming back from the current one. We need to start parsing some data for our presentation. Look for anything that's showing a decline that we can grab onto."

Sarcos turned to Representative Jeffries, "Joey, let's you and I go talk with your polling team and work on the wording for the next poll. They're not giving us what we're going to need for Congress if we want to keep this in pharma's hands."

"Bea, Ed will take you to the hotel at five. We'll pick you up from there at 6:30 for dinner reservations at eight. Put something conservative on. We're going to be on display since we're eating with Joey and Representative Thomas. They always garner attention when we eat on the hill."

"Will do, but aren't we a couple hours away from DC?" Bea asked, making a mental note to not wear the backless dress that she had thrown into her suitcase "just in case" and to stick with the navy dress and pearls.

"We'll take the jet and have time to spare," Bill gloated. "Be in the lobby at 6:30."

Vinnie took Bea to the secondary lab at Gelinex Pharmaceuticals. As state-of-the-art as their Colorado lab was, even the secondary lab of Gelinex's made hers look like child's play. From a wall of extraction machines to multiple chromatography units, you could see your reflection in every piece of polished stainless steel in the massive room. Vinnie waved over a middle-aged man with glasses wearing a starched white lab coat.

"You must be Bea," he said, holding out his hand to meet Bea's. "Steve. Steve Lyons."

"Pleased to meet you. I hear we have some data to go over."

"That we do. Right this way," Steve pointed her towards the conference room on the back side of the lab.

"What way are we going?" he turned to ask Vinnie.

"Against, today. We need to focus on the Ways and Means Committee testimony," Vinnie replied.

"Chinese oil, it is."

Chapter 6

Bea walked through the lobby of the hotel and into the waiting elevator. Sheila had taken care of her check-in and had a begrudging Ed bring her luggage to her room earlier in the day. The few moments in the elevator were the first of her being alone since boarding the plane early that morning. She leaned up against the glass wall and let out a big sigh. Her day had felt like an episode of *The Twilight Zone*, and she was not looking forward to dinner – or the flight on the private jet. What she really wanted was a long bath and a good nap – and to snuggle with Izzie.

"Izzie!" she thought and grabbed for her phone to call Jaime and get an update. The door to the elevator opened and she stepped out – and into the chest of a very large man.

"So sorry!" Bea said before looking up to see the face of the body she had just collided with. "I know you," she said quizzingly as she made eye contact with the man that she had seen earlier that day behind the plain wooden desk at the office that morning. "What are you doing here?" she asked, noticing the bulge from the revolver under his sport coat.

"Just making sure you got here safe and sound. We haven't properly met. Mitch," he said offering his hand.

"Bea. So, am I safe and sound?" she asked, realizing that the Twilight Zone portion of her day was obviously not quite over yet.

"Yes, you are. And I'll be sure to keep you that way while you're here."

Bea squared her shoulders again and . . .

"IT'S RAINING MEN, HALLELUJAH! IT'S RAINING MEN!" her phone sang as she quickly hit the volume down button on her phone. Glancing at the screen, she saw Jaime's name. "I have to get this," she told the hulking Mitch as she walked quickly towards her room while answering the call.

Mitch chuckled, shook his head and entered the elevator. Bea looked back as she opened the door to see the elevator doors close with Mitch inside.

"Bea? You there?" Jaime asked.

"Yes, I'm so sorry. I'm here. I'm just now getting to my hotel room. How's Izzie? And you – how are you and Rufus?"

"We're all fine. Izzie hasn't had a seizure since last night and is eating and enjoying her time as greeter at the clinic."

"Greeter? Izzie? That I'd like to see!"

"We had to give her the job. She was running up to the door to greet everyone when they came in, so we figured we may as well make it official while she's here."

"That's hysterical – I really would love to see that!"

"I'll text you a pic later tonight."

"Thank you! That would be great!"

"So, how's the business trip going?"

"Enlightening," Bea said in a terse voice.

"That doesn't sound good," Jaime replied.

"Yeah, it's been interesting, to say the least. By the way, the CBD that you're giving Izzie. Where's it from?"

"We get it from a local grower/extractor. He's been making tinctures for us for a few years now. Why?"

"Just curious. I've heard that there are some oils in the market coming in from overseas that aren't very good."

"That may be the understatement of the year – especially if it's coming from China. China uses hemp for ground remediation and then sells the oil extracted from it over here – filled with heavy metals. They could use it for hempcrete or plastics and be just fine, but the big money is in CBD. So, they make a killing off a waste product for themselves and our government welcomes it with open arms. It's out there in products being sold in gas stations across the country.

Jaime continued, "People see CBD on a label and think they're getting something healthy when they're more than likely doing more harm than good by taking it if it's coming from overseas. We need regulation, but we need it done the right way."

"I guess the FDA needs to crack down on it."

"That's a tricky subject. Yes, the FDA needs to regulate it, but as a dietary supplement. We don't want them scheduling it so that it gets locked up with big pharma. That's the worst thing that could happen."

"Why would that be bad?"

"First of all, because it's a safe substance. There is no risk of overdose with CBD, no addiction and only a handful of contraindications with medication. It's a very safe cannabinoid and needs to be used in conjunction with other cannabinoids and terpenes for the best effect. Pharma understands single molecule medicine. They can't wrap their heads around full plant medicine. The results from the synthetic products that they've been producing to mimic cannabinoids have come with terrible side effects to the patients – and then they try to say that the side effects are from the cannabinoids rather than their synthetic versions. David Dawkins says it's like comparing an apple picked from a tree to a plastic apple. Eating a natural apple is healthy – eating a plastic one is going to cause problems. Scheduling CBD would be a blatant repayment from politicians to their pharma campaign donors. Plain and simple."

"Plain and simple may be a bit of an oversimplification, but I can see how you can come to that conclusion."

"It's not an oversimplification. Pharma sees a money-maker and wants the monopoly on it. It's all about profit – and about not LOSING the profit that they currently make on drugs that can be replaced by cannabinoids which are much safer and cheaper.

"Look at insulin," Jaime explained. "The cost of insulin – which these companies had absolutely NO money wrapped up in for R&D – has skyrocketed for no reason other than profit. And they need to keep bringing in that profit to keep stockholders happy. CBD and a handful of other cannabinoids have the opportunity to significantly reduce insulin dependence, if not completely wipe it out. That's a real threat to their bottom line, and that's just one treatment. Throw in Crohn's Disease, pain control, epilepsy, anxiety – and look at the studies coming out for Alzheimer's, cancer and immune diseases – and the entire pharmaceutical industry is in danger. I'm not saying that pharma shouldn't be studying it and using it in formulations, I'm just saying that they shouldn't be the only ones that can.

"It's a safe product," Jaime insisted. "Endocannabinoids are naturally made by your own body, and their phytocannabinoid equivalents are just as safe as the ones your body makes. There is no valid reason to schedule any part of the hemp or cannabinoid plants. None," Jaime said emphatically.

"I. . . I'm sorry. I didn't mean to get you upset."

"No, it's alright. There's a lot of misinformation out there and I just get worked up when greed takes precedence over the health of people – and their pets. Sorry, I didn't mean to unload on you like that. You were just asking a question; it's not like you're a part of that. You're just looking after Izzie."

"Yeah, just looking after Izzie," she said, her voice trailing off.

"You OK? I'm sorry I came on so strong. I just believe that there is a huge lack of integrity in the world right now and it seems to be contagious. I really didn't mean to dump all of this negativity on you. I'll make it up to you when you get back. I'll take you to one of my favorite spots – very peaceful and out of the way. You'll love it there, and so will Izzie."

"That would be wonderful, but there's no need to apologize. I get it. I'm just a little tired and I have to get ready for a dinner meeting in D.C."

"D.C.? I'm really going to have to find out what kind of research you do – without you having to kill me, that is."

"It's just boring stuff- just a lot of data to deal with. I'd really like to keep talking, but I have to start getting ready. Can I call you later tonight?"

"Let's just talk tomorrow. You don't need to be thinking about me or Izzie tonight. She's in good hands. You take care of business and give me a call when you get back tomorrow and we'll take it from there. Deal?"

"Deal. And thank you again for everything."

Chapter 7

Bea stepped off the elevator and into the lobby at 6:20, ten minutes before her appointed time to be picked up for dinner. She was tense as she had never been on a private jet before, nor had she been to dinner with politicians, and really would have preferred to be not doing either after the events of the day.

"You just really don't relax, do you?" a voice behind her asked.

Bea jumped and swirled around to see Mitch standing behind her, wearing the same sport coat with holster beneath it.

"Jesus! What are you doing here?" Bea asked, trying to catch her breath.

"Making sure you're safe and sound," replied Mitch.

"From who? From what? What do I have to be kept safe from?"

"Relax. It's just an expression. You're new to the city and we just don't want you going to any dangerous areas."

"Like your office this morning?"

"Exactly, but Ed and I both had eyes on you the entire time. That's our neighborhood and nothing happens there that we don't know about. We just like to make sure that our guests are taken care of. And you're a special guest."

"How so?"

"You just are. And tonight's a very special night. You'll be traveling in style to dinner in a Gulf Stream, picked up in a limo and whisked off to an amazing meal at Komi. It's a night you won't soon forget."

Bea just stared at him, emotionless and unimpressed. She couldn't care less about the plane, limo or restaurant. She was already extremely uncomfortable with what she had witnessed that day. While she was not sure if anything being done was illegal, she was confident that it was unethical. Now, with the extravagant activities of the evening, she felt like she was being paid off.

"Let's just get this over with." Bea muttered, walking towards the door.

"Most women would be thrilled with an evening like this."

"I'm not 'most women.' I'm a scientist," Bea proclaimed, flinging the door open into the side of the doorman.

"I'm so sorry! Are you okay? Can I get you some ice?"

"No, I'm fine, Miss," laughed the doorman. "But you'd better be careful tonight," he said, looking at Mitch with a wink. "She's a bit feisty!"

"That she is," Mitch agreed, leading her towards his car to take her to the private airstrip. "That she is."

Bea, along with Mitch, Dr. Sarcos and the rest of the crew, arrived at Ronald Reagan Washington National Airport and deplaned from the Gulf Stream. The plane was very nicely put together, but nothing overly extravagant. It was furnished with leather seats and couches, nice wooden tables, plush carpet and a wet bar, as well as a flight attendant to cater to everyone's needs. The flight was uneventful and quite boring for Bea as she was subject to the reminiscing of six middle-aged men reliving their youth.

"You're with me," Mitch said to Bea, pointing to an "understated" bright yellow Ferrari. "The guys need to talk business in the limo. We'll meet them there."

Bea checked out the inside of her eye sockets with an eye roll from hell and followed Mitch to the car. He opened the door and she lowered herself into the sports car – grateful that her dress had a full skirt rather than a pencil skirt, otherwise getting out of the car would be tricky, and possibly revealing.

"Overcompensating?" she muttered under her breath, referring to the flashy sportscar.

"Want to find out?" he challenged.

"That's a hard no."

Mitch got into the car, started the engine and drove – slowly, as to not get another sarcastic comment from his passenger – towards the exit. As they made their way onto the backroads towards the restaurant, he quietly asked, "So, what happened to you to make you this bitter?"

"I'm sorry, what?"

"I'm not trying to be confrontational, but you're an attractive, intelligent woman with a lot going for herself. But you're always on guard. Someone had to do something for you to act this way."

"Nothing happened. There's no hidden drama from my childhood or a lover that jilted me. What there is, however, is a revealing of parts of the business that I was not aware of when I joined the company and I really don't know how I feel about that. But I'm a professional and I will continue to act as one and fulfill my responsibilities. I just need to get the full picture of what I've signed up for and I don't really have that as of yet."

"Ah, I see," Mitch said, drumming his fingers on the steering wheel nervously. He was silent for the remainder of the drive with the exception of his finger drumming.

"We're here," he said, pulling up to the restaurant set in a townhouse in an upscale part of the city. "They're waiting for you inside."

"You're not coming in?"

"No, I have some people to see while I'm here. I'll see you on the plane on the way back though."

"Do you want me to get you anything to eat for the plane ride back?" Bea offered.

"Hey, don't you get soft on me."

"You don't have to worry about that. Get out of here."

The yellow Ferrari sped off quickly down the street and into the night. Bea turned and walked up the stairs to Komi's entrance and could already hear the laughter of the men from the plane as she was greeted at the door by a nice young Greek gentleman who led her to the table. The congressman and, she assumed, his wife were seated to one side of Bill Sarcos along with another couple, and Vinnie and his date were on the other side. Bea was seated at the end of the table with Vinnie's "plus one" on one side and one of the men from the plane on the other. She still didn't understand who these other men were, or at least tried to convince herself that she didn't know who they were, and definitely was not asking.

A waiter appeared immediately with wine for Bea along with a glass of water. He explained that there would be 12 courses to their meal that evening along with wine pairings, and asked if she would like anything else to drink besides the water and wine. Her eyes must have looked like saucers because Vinnie's guest offered, "Don't worry, the courses are amazing but small.

You'll still be able to walk when you leave – unless they get you with the wine."

"Oh, thank you. I don't think I've ever had a 12- course meal before and I think I'd remember that," she replied. Bea thanked the waiter, saying that the wine and water would be more than enough.

"I'm Jessica," Vinnie's guest said.

"Bea," she replied. "It's nice to meet you. There's quite a group of us here. I'm surprised they didn't take up the entire restaurant."

"It's definitely their favorite place. The guys don't have to worry about being too loud here," she said as two waiters started belting out a Greek ballad in the kitchen. "It's a fun place and the food is amazing. You'll love it. Just eat slowly so you don't fill up too quickly. You'll want to leave room for dessert."

"Oh, boy," Bea wondered how much room she had in the bodice of her dress – again grateful for the full skirt over the tighter straight dress.

By the fifth course, the conversation had died down and the food comas were starting to creep in. Talk at the table turned to business.

"Bea, did you get everything you needed from the lab today?" Sarcos asked.

"Just about. Steve is going to send me what we didn't have time to cover," she replied.

"Good. Follow up with him tomorrow afternoon. Let's make sure we have what we need to give the good congressman what he wants to include in the presentation for the hearing."

Just then, Bea's phone played a five second clip of "It's Raining Men." She grabbed the phone from her purse as everyone laughed uncontrollably.

"I'm so sorry! Please excuse me. It's a text from the veterinarian that's watching my dog. He's just sending photos of her to show me she's okay."

"Can I see?" Jessica asked.

"Yes, of course," Bea offered, showing her Izzie in her new role as greeter at the clinic.

"Adorable."

"Thank you. I'll just silence this." Bea held the phone in her lap, adjusting the notification volume down, while adjusting the main volume to maximum. She quickly hit the voice recorder button and then the home button to conceal the recorder, and placed the phone face down on the table, pretending to forget to put it back in her purse.

"I'm sorry. So, I'll get with Steve tomorrow afternoon to get the rest of the data from the Chinese oil study for what Representative Jeffries needs," she recapped.

"Yes, it's crucial that we glean the right information from the Chinese oil to show that CBD has more of a downside than a benefit. Then we'll switch over to the study on the Colorado oil for Vinnie so we can get these new drugs fast-tracked by the FDA," Sarcos explained.

"We have got to keep that data straight. Double and triple check everything in the report. The heavy metals from the Chinese oil will help us get what we need for Joey. It's diluted enough that we're getting great data showing that people's immune systems are being compromised, and we've even had a few come down with cancer. It's better than I hoped we'd be able to get." Sarcos turned to Vinnie, "That was genius, using a 15% oil for that. Just genius. Anyway," he said, focusing on Bea again, "Glean the bad from the Chinese oil and focus on that for the presentation. The Colorado oil will speak for itself. We won't have to look hard for the results on that oil – it's showing benefits we didn't even expect. By the way," he said, focusing his attention on the lady sitting next to Jeffries, "How are you feeling?"

"I feel like a new person," she answered, voice filled with excitement and gratitude. "I can't tell you the difference it's made, Billy. I have my life back."

"I'm so glad, Vicki. I know how hard it's been for you. I'm glad it's helping. It's great to see you back out and about. Joey didn't tell me we'd be seeing you tonight."

"We wanted to surprise you," Joey Jeffries said. "We wanted to see the look on your face when you walked in and saw her sitting here."

"It was a great surprise, you two! I'm so glad that it's making such a difference. But we have to keep that amongst us," Sarcos reminded them.

"I'm telling people that I switched medication and changed my diet," Vicki explained. "We've got it covered."

"Excellent, just excellent," Sarcos replied, genuinely happy for the improved health of his friend.

Just then, the waiter came by with another course and another wine to pair it with as the discussion at the table turned back to food and reminiscing. Bea took the opportunity to remove her phone from the table and return it to her purse to make room for another plate.

Chapter 8

Bea woke up early the next morning and caught her flight home. Dr. Sarcos agreed to let her work from home that afternoon since they had a late night with their colleagues the night before. As soon as she got off the flight and had boarded the train at the Denver airport, she called Jaime to check on Izzie.

"Izzie's phone, how may I be of assistance?" Jaime answered.

"Is it that bad?" Bea laughed, surprised at the butterflies in her stomach upon hearing his voice.

"Bad? It's an honor to serve royalty. Even Rufus has fallen into line. But in all seriousness, she's doing really well. Are you back in town?"

"Yes, I'm on the airport train right now. What does your schedule look like? I'd like to pick up Izzie when you have a minute free."

"How about I bring her over around 6:00 and I can go over a few things with you. Text me your address."

"Okay, 6:00 sounds good," she replied, trying to remember what state of disarray the house was in when she left. It was only yesterday morning but it felt like a week had passed. "I'll throw something together for dinner. Any preferences?"

"I'll eat just about anything, but don't go to any trouble."

"It's no trouble. I enjoy cooking - especially for people who'll eat just about anything."

"Sounds perfect."

"Great, it's a date. Wait, no . . it's a - um . . ."

"I'll see you around 6:00," Jaime replied, laughing as he hung up.

Just then the doors to the train opened and the mass of people moved towards the escalators, taking a mortified Bea in tow with them.

Bea got home and started cleaning immediately – scrubbing toilets, washing floors, doing laundry. By 5pm, she had changed the sheets, vacuumed the carpet and done the dishes. She glanced at the clock and decided to start dinner. She opened the fridge to see what her options were and it looked like cold cereal was going to be the best entrée she could offer based on the contents of the refrigerator and pantry.

Looking at the clock again, she had one hour to run to the store and make an impressive meal. Thank God for the Instant Pot! She settled on Tuscan Chicken Pasta and ran to Sprouts for some organic chicken and sun-dried tomatoes, along with the other handful of ingredients the recipe called for. She stopped by Blue Moon liquor on her way out and grabbed a bottle of red wine to pair it with.

Bea had everything prepped and ready to go when her phone rang – the screen read "Mum."

"Hi, Mum," Bea answered. "How are you feeling today?"

"Not too bad today. The weather's cooperating so I'm not feeling the aches as much today. How was your trip? I got your text about the corporate jet. Was it nice?"

"Yeah, it was okay. I thought it would be fancier, but it was cool. It was nice not dealing with the lines and mobs of people like I had on my commercial flight home. Ugh. Hey, can I call you later?" Bea asked. "The vet that's been watching Izzie is due to be here any minute. He's bringing Izzie home for me and I'm making dinner."

"Oh! The Doctor!!!!"

"Mum, really . . . "

"Of course, you can call me later. Enjoy your evening – with the hot doctor!!!!! Love you!"

"Love you too, Mum."

Bea hung up the phone and looked around the house. Pleased with how everything looked, she set the pressure cooker button on the Instant Pot to five minutes and returned the unused ingredients back to their homes. As long as Jaime didn't look in the closets, the impression should be a good one. Glancing at the time on the phone, she realized that he would be there any minute now and the butterflies in her stomach started flying around like they were caught in a windstorm.

"Nope," she told herself sternly. "We're not going there. This is NOT a date. It's a thank you dinner for watching Izzie and that's it. With some wine. And a cheesecake. Oh, and maybe some nice music. ALEXA – PLAY JAZZ MUSIC," she yelled at the cylinder on the table across the room.

"ALEXA – PLAY 70'S ALTERNATIVE ROCK," yelled Jaime from the screen door at the front of the house.

Startled, Bea knocked over the bottle of wine that she had opened to breathe and it started emptying itself all over the counter. "Crap," she squeaked grabbing a towel and righting the bottle.

"Everything okay in there? Can I come in?"

"Yes, please do. Sorry, I just knocked over the wine."

"Then it's a good thing I brought a bottle with me," Jaime replied as Izzie led him into the kitchen.

"Izzie!" Bea squealed happily, picking her up and hugging her. "Mommy missed you so much!" she continued, kissing her repeatedly.

"Wow, I hope someone misses me like that someday."

"Don't we all? And thank you so much for taking care of her. I so appreciate it! I don't know what I would have done without your help."

"It really wasn't any trouble. Miss Izzie is quite a little lady. I enjoyed my time with her."

"Where's Rufus?"

"I left him at home. I thought it would be a little less hectic if it were just the three of us tonight. I'll bring him some other time."

Bea blushed, thinking of the circumstances of "some other time" and then quickly regained her composure. "There's still half a bottle of wine that didn't end up on my counter. Can I offer you some?"

"That would be great," he replied, leaning in and kissing her on the cheek. "Mind if I take a look around?"

"Go right ahead," she replied. It was quite a feat to be able to speak as she had to pick her jaw up off the floor after the unexpected peck on the cheek. The butterflies in Bea's stomach were caught up in quite the windstorm and the kiss on the cheek had just ramped it up to a category 3 hurricane, leaving Bea a bit lightheaded. Izzie squirmed in her arms to get free of the tightening squeeze that her mom was inadvertently subjecting her to and finally barked to get her attention.

"Oh, sorry Izzie!" Bea quickly put Izzie on the floor and she scuttered off to the living room to resume her spot on her throne.

Bea poured a glass of wine, drank half of it, filled it again and poured a glass for Jaime, joining him in the living room.

"This is a beautiful house. How long have you been here?"

 "Almost a month." Bea handed him his wine. "I still have boxes in the garage to unpack, but it's coming along."

Jaime took the glass of wine and took a sip, looking at Bea over the rim of the glass while he did. She blushed and looked down at her glass, breaking eye contact as the hurricane in her stomach just hit a cat 4 rating.

"I may be a bit out of line here," he said quietly, in an almost bedroom voice, "but I think you're a remarkable woman and I'm hoping to get to know you a lot better. Is that okay with you?"

"I, um, yes, most definitely. I would like that very much."

"Can I kiss you?" he asked, taking the glass of wine out of her hand and putting the glasses on the table next to where Izzie was sitting, ignoring the two of them.

"Uh huh," was all Bea could get out as Jaime's eyes locked with hers.

Jaime put his arm around Bea and lightly brushed his lips against hers. "Are you sure?" he asked.

"Uh huh," she muttered again, catching her breath as the butterflies in her stomach were being battered about by a full-on category 5 hurricane that would destroy any city in its path. She stepped into him and put her hands on his chest, tugging gently at the fabric on his shirt as he kissed her, slowly running his hand up and down her back while his other arm held her tightly to him.

Bea put her arms around him, holding him close and melted into the kiss. They stood there, gently exploring each other until the Instant Pot chimed, letting Bea know that she needed to release the pressure (oh, BOY did she need to release the pressure) and stir in the remaining ingredients.

"Stupid thing cooks too fast," she thought to herself, offering Jaime a couple quick soft kisses before pulling herself away. "I'll be right back. I just have to finish something with dinner."

"Quite alright. We've got all night."

Bea jogged into the kitchen, did a quick release on the Instant Pot, removed the chicken from the pot and added the remaining ingredients. She quickly chopped the chicken and added it back to the pot, stirring to thicken the sauce.

"I hope you're hungry," Bea called to Jaime from the kitchen.

"It smells amazing," he replied. "What is it?"

"Tuscan Chicken Pasta," she said, taking the dishes out of the cabinet and carefully spooning the creamy chicken pasta dish with colorful bits of spinach and sun-dried tomato onto the square ecru dinner plates. She grabbed two forks and headed to the dining room.

Jaime grabbed the two glasses of wine and joined her. "That smells and looks incredible. If it tastes half as good as it looks, I may want seconds."

"Just make sure to leave room for dessert."

"That's right. I heard you saying something about cheesecake when I came to the door."

Bea's jaw again was agape, realizing he had heard the FULL conversation to herself in the kitchen earlier.

His eyes sparkled as he pulled back Bea's chair for her and pushed it forward as she sat at the cozy, square table for four. He sat at the side nearest her and rested his hand on her thigh.

"Thank you for cooking. This really does look amazing."

"I hope you like it."

Jaime and Bea talked for hours over dinner and he explained

Izzie's treatment plan and the science of how the CBD he was giving her prevents seizures. After the events of her business trip, she was beginning to understand more and more about the endocannabinoid system and how it works. She was grateful that Jaime was knowledgeable about the benefits and had tried it with Izzie – and even more grateful that it was working.

Bea cleared the table and poured the rest of the wine from the bottle that Jaime had brought into their glasses. He joined her in the kitchen, coming up behind her, wrapping his arms around the front of her and kissed her neck seductively. Bea turned around and kissed him back, forgetting about the dishes and everything else in the world other than him.

The kiss turned more and more passionate as their hands roamed each other's bodies, getting to know the curves and lines, inviting each other to learn more, explore more, want more.

Meanwhile, in the living room, Izzie had long grown weary of the two of them and had fallen asleep on her throne on the couch.

"Bea," Jaime whispered, "I either need to leave right now or we need to continue this in another room. I'm okay either way, but I really can't continue at this rate without losing my mind. It's your call and I'm good either way. I promise."

Bea grabbed her glass of wine in one hand and Jaime's hand in the other and led him down the hall to her room. There was no way she was letting him leave her in the state she was in. There was only one cure for what was ailing her, and it sure wasn't CBD.

Chapter 9

Bea woke up early, fed Izzie and gave her the CBD tincture, got dressed and headed out to work. Filled with a new-found energy, she arrived at the office an hour early and got straight to work.

Steve, the R&D director at Gelinex, had sent over the rest of the results on the Chinese oil study and Bea dove right in – but with a more skeptical view.

The CBD oil that they brought in from China came from hemp that was used to remediate the soil. She discovered that the hemp was grown in industrial areas where waste chemicals were released from manufacturing plants onto surrounding fields and then was tilled into the soil. With pollution levels being an issue in China, the manufacturing plants were shut down and moved to the coast. so the air pollution coming from the plants would be carried over the sea into South Korea rather than affecting their own population. This left large abandoned plants and the polluted land surrounding them open for innovation.

Scientists had long known about the ability of hemp to pull heavy metals from the earth and, in essence, heal the land. In earlier days, it was an integral part of crop rotation to keep the biome of the soil healthy, which helped produce healthier crops. And it worked very well with the polluted fields in China, while also producing a new product to export to the Americans – rather than selling the chemical-laden CBD oil to their own residents.

A great business model – heal the land (over many years of planting) and maximize the waste product (the harvested hemp) for profit. They could have used the harvested material for hemp paper, rope, clothing, plastic, biofuels, hemp-crete, insulation or a myriad of other purposes. But the highest return was in CBD oil. Until the Farm Bill of 2014 passed, the only CBD oil legally allowed to be sold in the US came from foreign soil. It was illegal to grow hemp in the states before then, which left the doors wide open for China. They found a hungry and uneducated market where they could dump their toxic product and cash in.

Yet even in this dirty, diluted oil, there was something to learn. Bea was looking for the common denominator beneath the layers, the hidden key. While that's not what Dr. Sarcos wanted her to find, it was her new driver. Yes, on the surface, the heavy metal-laden, watered down CBD oil was horrific and should never be put into any living being's body, but there was something else that was trying to be expressed just below the obvious.

The arsenic, lead, pesticides, mercury and other toxic pollutants were well known to be carcinogenic, in addition to being the root cause or contributing factor of a host of ailments, but the study only showed a fraction of a percent of the participants falling ill to them. There should have been a significant subset of participants experiencing toxicity-induced illnesses due to the chemical levels in the oil, but it simply wasn't the case.

Bea made notes in a notebook of her findings, careful not to put anything on her work computer. Somehow, the cannabinoids in the oil were helping the body protect itself from the harmful effects of the pollutants. She knew from the results of the Colorado oil that CBD and other cannabinoids helped alleviate symptoms of the participants – and balanced out blood sugar levels – by supporting and boosting the Endocannabinoid System (also known as the ECS).

It isn't that the cannabinoids are a magic substance, but rather they are the fuel for the ECS, which is like the wiring of a house that provides electricity where it is needed when a switch is turned.

The Endocannabinoid System is the body's internal highway through which messages are sent. Bea recalled that the Mayo Clinic referred to it as a distributed network of receptors and signaling molecules. A published study in The National Institute of Health's PubMed explained that neurons in our bodies use this signaling system to communicate with each other and that the activation of CB receptors (the receptors that work with cannabinoids) expressed by activated microglia (the macrophages of the brain) control immune-related functions.

It's the perfect internal "body-wide-web," rather than world-wide-web, where the immune, nervous and other systems in the body can post what they need and receive it efficiently. And even with the existence of toxic chemicals in the Chinese oil, the CBD – working together with other cannabinoids – was helping the body get the messages through to the immune system be able to counteract the ill effects.

"It explains so much," Bea thought to herself. "It's not the cannabinoids that are 'curing' everything. It's the ECS being fueled by the cannabinoids that is allowing the body to do what it does best – heal itself. No wonder the pharmaceutical companies are freaking out! Healthy people don't need expensive drugs, and stockholders demand returns on their investments."

"How is the presentation prep coming along?" Dr. Sarcos asked, standing in her office doorway.

Bea jumped at the sound of his voice, scattering papers across her desk.

"I didn't hear you come in." Bea gathered her notes and papers. "I'm compiling the information that Steve sent over. I should have a rough draft of the findings by this afternoon for you."

"Good. I want to have plenty of time to fine tune them for Jeffries. I'll be in my office if you have any questions. This project has priority over any other right now. You can use one of the Lab Rats if you need to."

"Thank you, I may do that," Bea knew that a full analysis of the oil from China detailing levels of every chemical and cannabinoid in the oil was going to be needed for her to better understand the findings beneath the obvious in this study, and had already asked Adam, the most promising of the Rats, to take care of that.

"Dinner tonight? My place – bring Izzie," read the text from Jaime. Bea's butterflies made a quick flutter to remind her of the previous evening's events.

"Most definitely!" she replied, excited to see him again and to see his place. Izzie had already slept in his bed more than once and Bea was feeling a little jealous of that. "Send the address?"

"On its way."

Bea got back to work on the presentation for the Ways and Means committee, detailing "The Dangers of Cannabidiol." Each keystroke increased her feelings of unease about what she was doing, now that she knew the science behind cannabidiol. She wondered how many people might choose not to research and try CBD because of the presentation that she was preparing with bad data.

While the data from the study supports their claims, the only reason it did was because of the use of highly contaminated oil. Knowing that they would also be submitting results from the pure CBD oil study to the FDA that would show strong benefits from its use made her conscience scream that much louder.

The more research she did, the more she thought about her mother and the handful of prescriptions she took daily for her fibromyalgia. She had seen some studies in PubMed that tied the ailment to the Endocannabinoid System (ECS) and wondered if it would help, but didn't dare mention anything at the office. From what she found, the combination of using a vape along with a strong tincture would be the best start for boosting her ECS. The tincture was a no-brainer, as it's a good solid methodology that's been used for a thousand years, with some improvements over time, of course. The vape part of the equation was trickier.

There had been a lot of backlash against the vape industry, and a lot of it was warranted. Non-CBD vapes were basically "cigarette-light" products with all of the chemicals, additives and nicotine added to attract and hook users. But there were some well-documented benefits in the efficacy and speed of the vape delivery method for CBD, and the CBD market – on average – approached their products with a more holistic viewpoint, stripping the contents down to natural ingredients and leaving out anything that was not critical to the effectiveness of the product for their customers. The two sides of the industry couldn't be more opposite – one side trying to ensnare customers with addictive chemicals and additives while the other side trying to help them with natural, safe and effective ingredients that studies have shown to be beneficial.

Bea would much prefer diving deeper into how to help her mother, but for now she needed to complete the draft and get it to Dr. Sarcos without feeling like she'd sold her integrity to the highest bidder.

Chapter 10

Bea and Izzie arrived at Jaime's house, a large ranch home on several acres. The front door was wide open. The girls were both greeted with a nose in the butt by Rufus. Izzie walked straight into the house to the overstuffed chair by the window and made herself comfortable while Rufus settled at the foot of the chair.

"You found the place," Jaime called out from the back of the house. "I'll be right there."

"The door was open. I hope it's okay that we let ourselves in."

"Of course it is," Jaime replied, walking towards Bea from the hallway. "You can let yourself in anytime," he said wrapping his arms around her. "Besides, the place already looks better with you in it."

Jaime kissed Bea tenderly and asked, "Hungry?"

"Uh huh," Bea nodded, not exactly sure what he was asking she was hungry for, but whatever it was, the answer was yes. And she definitely knew she was thirsty!

"Good, can I offer you a glass of wine?"

"That would be wonderful," she whispered back, getting more and more excited about being at his home. "Your place is lovely. You have an amazing view of the foothills."

Jaime walked to the kitchen and returned with a bottle of Merlot and two glasses. He walked over to the couch and set them on the table, motioning for her to join him. He poured two glasses, handed her one and touched his glass to hers. Looking into her eyes, he said, "To amazing views."

Jaime sat on the couch and put his arm out for her to sit next to him and wrapped it around her. She instinctively leaned into him and rested her head on his shoulder. He leaned in towards her and kissed her as she melted into his body. She was right. She was hungry – and this was exactly what she was hungry for.

Jaime started preparing dinner as Bea napped in his bed. He was cooking his go-to meal that he had cooked a hundred times before – tenderloin steak on the grill and garlic asparagus in the skillet. It was a delicious meal that he had mastered years ago, and he was sure that it would impress Bea. As he prepared the grill, Rufus & Izzie followed Jaime closely, hoping that something would fall from his plate while he was cooking.

It was a gorgeous evening with the weather in the low 70's and just enough of a breeze to make the windchimes sing. Jaime's back patio was well suited for guests. The sprawling flagstone area was arranged with a dining area, a living area complete with couch, chair and low table, and a few chaise lounges and hammocks hanging from various trees that surrounded the patio. The centerpiece, however, was a stone firepit surrounded by sets of double-wide cushioned chairs with ottomans.

Along one of the walls was Jaime's favorite part of his home – an outside kitchen, complete with grill, smoker, running water, refrigerator and a brick pizza oven. He used it as often as possible while he enjoyed his unencumbered view of the open space that led up to the foothills.

"There you are," Bea said as she walked out onto the back patio. "Wow, this space is amazing." Bea took in the spacious patio and surrounding nature.

"I'm glad you like it," Jaime walked to her and kissed her. "Did you get a good nap?"

"Yes," she said shyly. "I guess I was just a little worn out from the day."

"Or the evening. I have the steak on. We'll be eating in about 15 minutes. Can I get you some more wine?"

"Thank you, but I think I'll stick to water for now. I still have to drive home tonight and I have an early morning."

"Understood, but let me know if you have a change of heart."

"Speaking of a change of heart," Bea started, "I've been looking into CBD quite a bit since I talked to you last about it and was wondering if I could pick your brain a little."

"Sure, what do you want to know?"

"Geez, where to start? I think I have a basic knowledge of the endocannabinoid system and how it acts as a messaging system in your body."

"Okay."

"And I know about the endocannabinoids that our bodies naturally make and the plant equivalents, or phytocannabinoids."

"Good," he said, flipping the steaks.

"But how do you know you're not getting junk CBD since it's not regulated?"

"Well, that's the million-dollar question. There are bad actors in the industry who will throw a label on a bottle and call it a miracle drug just to make a buck. And that's why it's important to know your source - know the company, know where the oil is coming from, where it's grown and under what conditions. Know who's doing the extraction, review the Certificate of Analysis, talk to the company and ask questions. You'll know if they're dodging the hard questions or if they're lying. And trust your gut if something doesn't seem right."

"That doesn't seem very easy for the common person to do," - even with her advanced degree in biochemistry, Bea wouldn't know where to go to get good oil if she hadn't had the test results from her own lab. "Can't COA's be manipulated?"

"Anything can be changed with the right software these days, but it's pretty hard to fake a relationship with a customer. You're either knowledgeable or you're not.

"Several years ago," Jaime began, "I started listening to podcasts and ran across a really good one - CBD Talk Podcast. They have some interesting guests from within the industry – scientists, extractors, growers, manufacturers. The information in the interviews help me fill in some areas around where I still have questions about CBD. The guests regularly give out their contact information on the show and welcome people to contact them and ask questions. That would be my first recommendation – listen to CBD Talk Podcast. They're on Spotify, iTunes, Google Play – the majors.

"But one guy in particular," he continued, "is one of the hosts on the podcast, Harley Damico. He's in Pennsylvania now where he has started growing hemp. He has a company called **Homegrown Essentials** and has a line of vape products that I really like – all natural, no chemicals added. It's all about the terpenes and the synergy between them and the cannabinoids. So, I guess I started growing my knowledge base from there in addition to people that I know locally. Now I know people across the country that I can pick up the phone and call if I have a question about anything."

Jaime continued, "So, I guess my answer would be to utilize your friends' knowledge if you have people in the know – which you do – or jump in somewhere and start asking questions – and listen to podcasts – specifically ones that aren't just selling their product - to get to know some of the people in the industry. The ones who are in it for the right reason will take your calls and answer your questions – whether you buy from them or not."

"Do you think I could talk to Harley?" Bea asked.

"Of course. What's up?"

"I'm just worried about my mom. She has fibromyalgia and I hate that she's always in so much pain. If there's a chance that she can get any relief at all from CBD, then I want to get her on it. "

"Wow, that's tough. I've heard good things about CBD and fibromyalgia. I think you have a good shot at giving her some relief, if not helping her body get rid of that completely. I would actually go at this two ways – a vape and either a tincture or a gel cap if you don't think she'd take a tincture. Some people, especially older people, are more likely to be consistent with taking pills over the tinctures because they're used to that method and, like with medicine, taking it consistently is important - especially with a chronic illness."

"Let me give you Harley's info as well as another contact. It's hard to find anyone more knowledgeable about vapes and CBD in general than Harley. Vin Ciffa at **Clean Green Mart** has some great capsules and tinctures that are liposomal based that would be a good partner to Harley's vapes. The bioavailability in the liposomal products is a lot higher than in regular tinctures and that's key. My mom takes his stuff every day and it works wonders for her."

"What does she take it for?" Bea asked.

"She takes it mostly as a neuro-protectant and for anti–inflammatory properties rather than using NSAIDs, but it's also helping her with her sleep."

Jaime explained, "That's the thing with CBD that most people don't get. It's not about specific symptoms or illnesses, it's about supporting the endocannabinoid system so your body can send the internal messages more efficiently to heal itself. Most of us have a cannabinoid deficiency and our body can't get those messages through. It's like rush hour in Denver – but the traffic never ends.

"If the messages can't get through, small problems can turn into big problems, and then those problems turn into chronic and severe illnesses. Before you know it, you've got cancer and are throwing radiation at your body. Supporting your endocannabinoid system keeps those highways clear so the messages get through and your body can do what it's meant to do. That's why the body makes cannabinoids in the first place and has an endocannabinoid system. Sometimes the human body – or animal body like Izzie's - just needs a boost because our lifestyle - stress, diet, whatever – is draining us."

"Why isn't this information mainstream? Why doesn't everyone know about this?" Bea asked and then quickly answered her own question. "Money. Money and power."

"Those who have the money, have the power," Jaime answered,

"until enough people force change. When mothers of children with chronic illnesses – whose illnesses aren't being effectively controlled by drugs - find something that can control it, things start happening. When veterans find relief for symptoms that the VA and handfuls of drugs can't touch, things start happening. And," Jaime continued, wrapping his arms around Bea, "even when people find safer treatments for their Izzie's instead of giving them drugs with horrid side effects, things start happening.

"People start talking and thinking, which leads to studies; which lead to treatments; which lead to more people using it and more studies and more treatments and cures. The key is in doing studies because the science IS THERE, and the studies will show that. Replicable studies prove efficacy and the medical field WILL listen to science – but pharmaceutical companies are doing their best to make sure that doesn't happen. But when you have enough people talking about how it's helping them, and doctors listening to their patients over their pharma reps, things start happening.

"Politicians are starting to see the light and that's helping as well. Big pharma still owns a lot of them, but grass roots groups are starting to find them and point them out more and more – even with money hidden in PACs – and they'll get voted out. Choosing money over the health and well-being of your constituents is not a strong platform for re-election.

"Sorry, I didn't mean to go off on a tangent like that. You look like a deer caught in headlights. Let's just relax and eat and you can tell me about your day at work today," Jaime offered.

"Let's just relax and eat instead," Bea suggested. Her work was the last thing she wanted to talk about.

Chapter 11

Bea drove into work early, filled with both purpose and confusion. On one hand, she knew what she wanted to do – find a way to expose what Dr. Sarcos and Medicroy Labs are doing – but on the other hand she had no idea how to do that without losing her job and being sued because of the NDA. If she had known then what she knew now, she never would have signed it. But the lawyers knew what was going on, and the position it would put people in, and they wrote it with that in mind.

Bea would have gone to the news but they wouldn't understand the importance of what was happening. They were still stuck on doing stories about people hot-boxing or about people complaining of their neighbors smoking joints in their backyards and the smoke traveling into theirs. She couldn't go to the police because what they were doing wasn't technically illegal.

You see studies contradicting each other all the time, based on who is sponsoring it. One minute milk is bad for your health and the next minute it's doing your body good. Again, it's all about the money behind the message. Like with the Chinese oil, they pull whatever data suits their agenda from the results and focus solely on that. And now she was tasked with doing the same.

Bea was driving east on Harmony Road, directly into the rising sun, when her phone rang. She didn't recognize the number but instinctively answered it anyway, "Beatrice Clarke."

"Hey, it's Mitch," the voice on the phone answered. "Don't go into the office just yet. Meet me at IHOP instead. It's your next left. I'll be waiting for you there." Click.

"What the fuck?" Bea said out loud. It was 6:05 in the morning. What was Mitch doing in Colorado and how did he know she was on her way to the office, or more specifically the exact location of her car?

Bea took the next left and parked in the nearly empty lot at IHOP. She grabbed her phone and her purse and went inside to meet Mitch. Seated next to him was Jessica, Dr. Zambini's plus one at Komi's back in D.C. She paused for a moment and stared, confused, at the two of them. Then she made her way to the booth and sat across from them.

"What's going on?" Bea asked tersely, wanting to cut to the chase. She was already highly irritated that Mitch had been following her and had no clue as to why Jessica was there.

Mitch took the lead, "We need to know where you stand on the studies."

"Where I stand?"

"We're taking a big risk right now. We need to know where you stand."

"What in the literal fuck are you talking about? You've been following me – for God knows how long – and now you're asking me where I stand on the studies and saying YOU'RE taking a big risk? What in the hell are you talking about? And why are you here?" she asked Jessica.

"We want to tell you," Jessica said calmly, her palms laid flat on the table in front of her, "but we need to know your feelings about the studies and what is happening at the lab first. We know you're friends with Jaime, and he's . . ."

"YOU FOLLOWED ME TO JAIME'S HOUSE?" Bea yelled.

"Please, please keep your voice down," Jessica said, glad that there was only one other patron there so early in the morning. "I will explain everything. We just need to know where you stand on what's happening at Medicroy."

"No, you're not getting any information from me until I know what's going on," Bea snapped back, furious at what was happening and wondering what else they knew about her and her whereabouts.

Jessica looked at Mitch, and Mitch nodded reluctantly to Jessica. "We're taking a big chance here, but we already think we know where you stand based on, well, you spending time with someone who is a big proponent of CBD."

"I haven't told him anything, if that's what you're worried about. I haven't broken your precious NDA," Bea shot back.

"No, we weren't suggesting that. That's not why we're here.

It's just the opposite," Mitch joined in. "We want to help you break it. We know how to break it."

"Seriously, stop talking around the subject. WHAT are you doing here and what is this all about?" Bea demanded.

"We are reporters for the Washington Post and are doing an expose on Medicroy Labs and their ties to the mafia, Congressman Jeffries and Gelinex Pharmaceuticals," Jessica answered. "And we need your help to do that."

Just then the waitress came up with a cup of coffee for Bea, "Two creams, two sugars – just how they said you liked it, sweetie. I'll be back in a bit with your order."

"You know how I take my coffee?" Bea asked accusingly.

"I remembered from the restaurant," Jessica explained. "You had a cup of coffee with dessert."

"OK, I'll give you that one," Bea said, accepting that explanation.

Mitch continued, "We've been working on exposing Sarcos for about six months. We got a tip from one of the interns at the congressman's office about what he overheard while working there last December under Representative Jeffries. He got in touch with us and I started working on getting a job as security with Gelinex about 3 months ago . . ."

"And I was able to find a way to meet Vinnie Zambini and,

well, get close to him to get some information as well," Jessica explained. "Mitch and I both have a lot to lose by talking to you about this, but we think we know the type of person you are. You seemed to be very much in conflict with what you learned while you were in Virginia. We're hoping you can help us bring this to light. We're also presenting at the Ways and Means committee, after Congressman Jeffries. Well, not us but NORML – the cannabis activist organization. We want to be able to present the other side of the data that he's giving including the data from the Colorado oil as well."

"Are you crazy? I will lose my job! They will sue me for everything I have, and even everything I don't have!" Bea argued.

"You'll definitely lose your job," Mitch stated, "but they won't be able to sue you. We've given Medicroy's NDA to NORML's legal team and they have found a loophole and will defend you in any suits brought against you. They said that there is no way that the NDA will hold. It was written to scare you, that's all. I have a written offer from them to represent you if it comes to that, in exchange for the information and your testimony, under oath, to the Ways and Means Committee."

Jessica offered, "Look, I know this is a lot being thrown at you right now, and we know we're asking a lot from you. We're asking you to give up a very lucrative job. But we also know that you know what you're contributing to and the damage that a study with malicious intent can do. It can set back progress for years and tip the scales to the pharmaceutical companies. It could literally cost lives that could have been saved by cannabinoid-based products. We're not asking for your answer right now. We just want you to think about it."

Just then, the perky "morning-person" waitress returned with a bag for Bea, "I believe yours was to go? Blueberry muffin, two egg bites and an apple for later." She smiled, placed the bag on the table and went back to the kitchen.

Bea just stared at the bag, then at Mitch and Jessica. She stood up, took the bag and walked back to her car, as if in a trance. The last ten minutes were a complete blur to her. She got into her car and drove to work completely baffled by what had just transpired and what she was going to do with all of this information. But before she did anything, she knew she needed to get some of that Colorado oil to her mother.

Bea was able to get into the lab before anyone arrived. Dr. Sarcos was in Denver all morning meeting with his supplier so he wouldn't be in for hours. She retrieved two bottles of the Colorado oil from the lab and left one at Adam's workstation with a note to give a full breakdown of all components in the bottle. Adam was one of the Lab Rats who showed a lot of potential. He asked a lot of questions – questions that Dr. Sarcos did not appreciate and could possibly get Adam fired. She put the second bottle of the Colorado oil in her purse and would ship it to her mother at lunch.

Bea went to her office, pulled out her phone and went to **ehomegrown.com** - Harley's site that Jaime had given her for vape products – and chose the 500mg terp-infused cartridge kit to pair up with the tincture. If she sent off the tincture today, they should both arrive at the same time. She knew it wouldn't be hard to get her mom to use them, as she would try anything to get rid of her symptoms. She wondered how much pain she could have avoided for her mother if she would have had an open mind at the time, but she was going to try to make up for that now.

For the next couple hours, Bea worked on the revisions for the Ways & Means presentation for Dr. Sarcos while also taking notes in her notebook on how CBD was countering the effects of the toxic components of the oil they had used in the study. She sketched out graphs of the results of exposure to the separate chemicals from known studies and added data from their study. The graphs showed the results of their study illustrating the reduction in harm experienced by the participants when CBD was added to the toxic chemicals the participants were ingesting. If she did decide to cooperate with Jessica and Mitch, that was the information she wanted to get across.

Bea heard a knock on her open office door and looked up to see Adam standing there with the data she had requested. Adam was, by far, her favorite Lab Rat and she did her best to shield him from Sarcos, telling him to go directly to her with any questions rather than bring them to Sarcos. While he didn't know what angle the studies were taking from the information that was coming from the lab, the benefits of CBD jumped right off the paper and, figuratively, slapped him in the face. He was very excited by the science that was showing clear benefits in using CBD and the unrivalled safety of the compound.

Adam had ideas on how to maximize the oil and which terpenes were effectively boosting the minor cannabinoids in the formulation. Dr. Sarcos' pat answer to him was to "stay in your lane" - that Adam had no clue what he was talking about, that anything he learned in the lab belonged to the lab due to the NDA he signed, so he should stick to doing what he was told.

"I have the results that you asked for. I had already done this on my own last week because I was curious. Please don't tell Dr. Sarcos." Adam handed Bea a binder with the cannabinoid, terpene and chemical breakdown of the oil that was sourced from China.

"Don't worry – your secret's safe with me. But I wouldn't mention it to the others."

"Not a chance. Did you see the effect that the CBD had on mitigating the harm that the chemicals did to the rats? I'm assuming that you were using rats – or were you using some other animal? Either way, it's awesome. And that was just with a weak concentration of CBD. So, I added some of the Colorado oil in there and ran an analysis and it really showed the potential benefits – good stuff."

Adam showed Bea the printouts and graphs that he had created based on the results that he had gotten from his testing.

"Close the door," Bea told Adam.

"Huh?"

"Please, close the door."

Adam looked quizzically at Bea, reached behind him and closed the door.

"Adam, do not show this to anyone. It could get you fired."

"I won't – I know better. Dr. Sarcos has made it abundantly clear that he doesn't want me to do anything other than the tasks he gives me. There's no chance I'd show him this."

"Did you prepare this data on the company laptop?"

Adam's face went white and he stared at Bea.

"Get me your laptop – NOW!"

Adam ran back to the lab and returned to Bea's office with the laptop, closing the door behind him. Bea knew that IT scheduled backups of data every evening and that they would have it on their server by now but IT didn't likely rummage through the files of the Lab Rats' computers. She opened the laptop and grabbed a thumb drive from her purse.

"Where's the file?" she asked Adam.

Adam went to the folder where he had stored everything. Bea copied the information onto her thumb drive, opened the individual files in his folder, deleted the content and copied and pasted old recipes, notes and blog posts from her thumb drive in its place. Deleting the files from the laptop would be a red flag that IT would pick up on but changing the data in the file was less likely to get noticed – especially if the file size didn't change significantly.

"Give me your personal email address and I'll send these to you tonight but don't EVER put anything like this on your work laptop again."

"I won't – I promise," Adam replied, realizing that there was more to what was going on at Medicroy Labs than met the eye. "What's going on? I mean, why is Dr. Sarcos so against us compiling data like this?"

"At this point, the less you know, the better, but I will fill you in when the time is right. For right now, just keep your head down and your mouth quiet until I can answer your questions. You'll need to trust me on this."

"I do. You've always looked out for me. I won't put anything in my laptop from now on."

"Here," Bea handed him a blank journal from her drawer. "Put your notes in here and keep it in your satchel. Just be careful when you do it – you don't want to raise any suspicions. If they see the reports that you just handed me, you'll be fired on the spot. They don't want to see the benefits coming from CBD. Just trust me on this."

Chapter 12

The rest of the week was filled with more research, reviewing data and finalizing the presentation for Dr. Sarcos and Congressman Jeffries. The more she looked at the data from the Chinese oil, the more she saw just the opposite of what Sarcos wanted to present. When she talked to him about it, he was pleased with the data and suggested it be used as the basis for a study for Gelinex to support the FDA filings for their new line of cannabinoid-based drugs that they were submitting.

"This man has no conscience," Bea thought to herself as she drove home Friday evening. Between the notes from the Chinese oil that she had compiled and the reports Adam gave her, Bea had two notebooks filled with good data that, hands down, would show any science-driven person the non-debatable benefits of CBD, yet she was contributing to a presentation to declare just the opposite. Not that the data was not factual, but it was not complete – purposely omitting other data to support Medicroy's agenda. It was easy to use heavy metal, chemical-laden, low concentration CBD oil and cherry pick data to show that – on the surface – people were worse off when they used that specific oil. But when you looked at the full results that contained the complete breakdown of the tincture – complete with pesticides, lead, mercury and other heavy metal contamination – the fact that these people didn't end up in the hospital was a feat in itself.

Adam was right to think that the study was on rats, because no self-respecting scientist would give that concoction to a human. But Dr. Sarcos was definitely not self-respecting, and neither were the lawyers that drew up the consent forms for the study participants – the majority of whom were homeless and needed the money, damn the consequences.

"I can't do this," she said aloud. "Hey Google, call Mitch."

"Calling Mitch," her phone dutifully replied.

"Anthony Barret," the voice on the phone answered – a familiar voice.

"I'm sorry, I must have the wrong number," Bea said, about to hang up.

"Bea?" the voice said. "Bea, sorry – it's Mitch. Well, it's Anthony, but it's Mitch from Gelinex."

"Of course," Bea replied, frustrated at another layer of secrets being revealed.

"I'm sorry I didn't tell you the other day. I couldn't use my real name with Gelinex. There was too much of a chance that they might have checked up on me and realized that I was a journalist. Have you thought about our conversation?"

"Yes, and I want to talk with you and Jessica about – wait. I'm guessing that's not her name either. Right?"

"Correct. It's really not that uncommon for journalists to have aliases," he tried to explain. "It's easier to get to the truth if you become somebody who your subject relates . . ."

"Stop. Don't mansplain this shit to me. I'm not in the mood. I was lied to. That's what it comes down to. But I do want to talk to you and, whoever . . ."

"Melissa."

"Melissa about what's going on. When can you meet?"

"Hang a right at Lemay and I'll have Melissa meet us at Domenic's. They've got a Bolognese that will knock your socks off."

"Are you ever NOT following me?" she screamed into the phone and hung up. As much as the situation irritated her, a good Bolognese was hard to say no to, and a bottle or two of red wine to wash it down with would be the perfect end to her day. Izzie would be fine for a couple hours now that Bea had a doggie door installed and a time-released dog feeder. No more worries about not being home in time for her to go potty and feed her.

Bea turned into the parking lot at Domenic's and walked through the patio seating toward the front door with Mitch/Anthony catching up behind her. She went directly to the bar, put her purse on the counter and ordered, "Purple Haze martini, please."

"I'll have a Negroni," Anthony ordered, walking up to the bar beside her. "We're waiting for a third."

"Coming right up. Came back for the Bolognese, right?" the bartender asked Anthony.

"You know it," Anthony laughed.

Bea stared straight ahead while sitting at the bar and said, "You know I'll lose my job."

"I know."

"You know the industry will blackball me for being involved with Medicroy."

"I didn't think you cared that much about the industry or what it thought," Anthony sipped his Negroni.

"It's hard NOT to care when you see the science behind what they're fighting for." Bea drank half of her Purple Haze martini in one gulp, the blackberry liqueur soothing her worry.

"I don't know that you'll be blackballed. I think, with an explanation and recommendation from NORML, it could be just the opposite. You'll be exposing a coordinated effort by a pharmaceutical company to discredit CBD and then promote the scheduling of the same substance for its own financial benefit. That's not something that will be overshadowed by a few months of you working there without knowing what was going on."

Bea downed the rest of her drink and signaled to the bartender for another. The bartender looked wide-eyed at Anthony who shrugged his shoulders at the bartender.

"If you help us, you will have the public backing of NORML to defend you breaking your NDA and you will also be included as a co-author – with your approval – in the article that shows how you helped to expose them. We will support you 100% in any way we can."

"The study with the Chinese oil is basically poisoning people," Bea stated, still looking straight ahead, starting on her second martini. "They're purposely using hemp from heavy-metal soil remediation in China to make the tincture. It's full of lead, mercury, arsenic – terrible stuff. And their participants in the study are all homeless people." Bea polished off her second Purple Haze Martini as Melissa walked through the door.

Alarmed at what Bea had just said, Anthony waved Melissa over hurriedly.

"Wait," he said to Bea as Melissa joined them. "You're saying that Medicroy is knowingly and purposely using hemp oil from hemp that was used in soil remediation from China which contains toxic contaminants in their study and dosing this to homeless people - in an effort to get them sick and then blame the adverse effects on the CBD?"

"Yup," she answered, the two hastily downed Purple Haze martinis now working their way through her system. "And barely enough CBD in it to do any good. At least, that's what they THOUGHT." Bea's voice was getting louder with the liquid courage pulsing through her body. "But I have data from the study they're NOT making public showing that even the small amount of CBD that's in there is warding off a lot of the ill effects of the crap in the oil – well for most of them, at least. There are a couple who are really sick. But we could see from the pre-trial physical that their immune systems were already weak."

By this time, Melissa was on the opposite side of Bea, looking at Anthony with concern.

"Another one, please," Bea asked the bartender.

"Hey," Melissa jumped in, distracting Bea from ordering another drink so quickly. "I'm really hungry. How about we get a table and some appetizers? Their crab cakes and bruschetta are awesome."

"Yeah," Anthony chimed in, helping Bea from her seat. "Gotta save some room for the Bolognese as well."

Anthony made eye contact with the bartender, shook his head and mouthed "No" to the bartender as they moved to the high-top table behind them.

Anthony helped Bea into the chair next to the wall and sat beside her with Melissa across from her. The waitress came over promptly with menus and introduced herself.

"Hi, I'm Sandy and will be serving you tonight. I see you've already got your drinks from the bar, can I interest you in some appetizers?"

"Yes, I ordered a Purple Haze," Bea blurted out.

Melissa discreetly shook her head "No" to the waitress. "Can we get an order of bruschetta and an order of crabs cakes, please? And three waters?" Melissa requested, pulling a notebook and a pen from her bag to take notes.

"Hey," offered Bea, Purple Haze coursing through her body now, "let me get MY notebook out too!" Bea struggled with her bag, pulling out her glasses, her wallet, a pencil bag filled with pens, a bra, a water bottle, her laptop, a pair of socks, more pens and finally her notebook. She shoved everything but her glasses, a pen and her notebook back into her bag, put her glasses on and opened her notebook.

"Here's the breakdown of the China soil remediation oil tincture that they used for the study with the homeless people. It's TERRIBLE. I can't believe this can be legal to use, but they have waivers from everyone they gave it to. I have copies of everything on my thumb drive. Where is that?" she asked herself, grabbing her bag again, this time dumping all of the contents on the table.

"OK then, I guess THIS is happening," Anthony said, backing away from the table as a tampon from her bag rolled his way.

"How many drinks did she have?" Melissa whispered across the table as Bea rummaged through the contents of her bag, strewn across the table.

"Two – but two martinis in less than three minutes. And they don't skimp on the alcohol here."

"Apparently not," Melissa replied, leaning down to pick up items off the floor that Bea had accidentally pushed off the table. As she got back up, she glanced outside.

"Oh, shit." Melissa saw three men walk up the sidewalk and seat themselves in the patio area just outside the door to the restaurant.

Anthony turned around and immediately saw what caught Melissa's eye – Sarcos and Vinnie settling in at a table on the patio along with another gentleman that he didn't recognize.

"I found it!" Bea exclaimed, clueless as to what was happening just outside the front door of Domenic's. "I found it!"

"That's great," Melissa replied to Bea, while keeping an eye on Sarcos and company. "Let me help you put all of this back in your bag."

"OK," Bea giggled, completely overtaken by the six ounces of hard liquor she downed not even ten minutes prior that was now throwing a rave in her body – complete with glow sticks and techno music.

Melissa started moving the contents of the table back into Bea's bag, which Bea was trying desperately to hold open. Anthony had turned back around and looked at Melissa with well-founded concern on his face when Sandy, the waitress, came over with their appetizers.

"Yay! Food!" exclaimed Bea. "I haven't eaten a thing since breakfast!"

"Well, that explains a lot," noted Anthony.

"What are we going to do?" Melissa quietly asked Anthony.

"I'm not sure, but this is not good. Especially in the state that Bea is in."

Oblivious to what was happening around her, Bea gleefully sampled the bruschetta and crab cakes. "Aren't you guys going to have any?" she offered.

"No, you go ahead and eat it," replied Melissa, distracted by the unfolding issue of Sarcos and Vinnie sitting less than 30 yards away.

"Okay," exclaimed Bea happily. IT'S RAINING MEN suddenly blurted from the bowels of Bea's immense bag.

"Jaime!" Anthony blurted out, looking at Melissa who already knew what he was thinking.

"Jaime," Bea cooed, sounding like an audible heart emoji.

Melissa grabbed Bea's bag and searched frantically for Bea's phone as Bea rocked back and forth in her chair, singing along to the ringtone.

"Got it!" Melissa exclaimed as she answered the phone. "Is this Jaime?" she asked, already knowing the answer as his name was on the screen.

"Yes, who's this?" Jaime asked, puzzled by the unknown voice answering Bea's phone.

"I'm a friend of Bea's."

"Is Bea okay?"

"She's, well, probably more than okay – at least for right now. But she's probably not going to be doing too well tomorrow morning if she has another drink," Melissa answered as Bea finished her song in the background.

"Really?" Jaime laughed. "Does she need some help?"

"Definitely," Melissa replied, a plan hatching in her head. "Could you come to Domenic's off Harmony and get her? The sooner the better."

"Is she that bad off? It's not even 6 o'clock – what time did you guys start drinking?"

"I'll explain it when you get here. We just need to get her out of here quickly. It's complicated but if you could come soon it would be greatly appreciated!"

"Okay, then. I'm on my way."

Anthony and Melissa looked at each other, worried but hanging onto Jaime as their ray of hope while Bea hungrily finished off the appetizers. Melissa looked over at Sarcos' table, glad that Billy and Vinnie had their backs to them while the third guy, whom she didn't know, was facing them. The waitress had gotten them their drinks and was now taking their orders. Jaime could not get there soon enough.

Melissa caught Sandy's attention as she came back in and ordered the antipasto salad, figuring the more food, the better for Bea. At the very least, it would keep her busy for a bit.

"Coming right up," Sandy replied, disappearing into the kitchen.

"We need a plan here," Anthony said quietly to Melissa.

"Hey, I didn't get to talk to Jaime," Bea complained. "Where's my phone?" she asked, grabbing her bag to search through.

"Jaime's on his way here to see you," Melissa replied in her kindest voice, not wanting to risk agitating Bea which would make matters even worse. "He's on his way right now to get you."

"Yay!" Bea exclaimed. "But why is he coming to get me? Aren't we eating here? I wanted to try the Bolognese. You said Dominatrix had the best Bolognese."

"Domenic's, not Dominatrix," Anthony corrected, trying not to laugh, as Sandy returned from the kitchen, "and they're out of the Bolognese right now," he said, looking at Sandy pleadingly while nodding to her. "So, we thought we'd all go somewhere else and talk."

"Uh, yeah," Sandy said cautiously, playing along for the moment. "We're fresh out of Bolognese. Is someone coming to pick you up? Can I help you get home?" she asked, not sure what was happening and wanting to make sure that Bea was okay and not in danger with the two others at the table.

"My boyfriend is coming," Bea replied gleefully. "He's so cute. He's the best boyfriend ever. I hope he knows this place because I want to come back here and get the Bolognese."

"Is this your first time here?" Sandy asked Bea, trying to assess the situation.

"Yes, I just moved here a little while ago. Mitch – I mean Anthony – suggested I come here so we could talk. He was following me in his car when I called him on my way home from work. He does that a lot." Sandy looked at Melissa and then Anthony.

"He follows you in his car a lot?" Sandy asked, holding a finger up to Anthony, not letting him get a word in.

"Yup, he and Jessica-Melissa have been following me for a while. And then they buy me food, and tonight they bought me alcohol, too!"

"I'll be right back," Sandy said, turning towards the kitchen.

"Wait," said Melissa, getting up to follow her. "I can explain."

"No, she's explained enough," Sandy snapped back, continuing into the kitchen to grab the phone.

"Her boyfriend is on the way, at least wait until he gets here before you do anything. We will stay at the table. We won't go anywhere. Here's my card," Melissa pulled her Washington Post business card from her pocket. "You can call my office and verify who I am. We're working on a story and things just got out of hand tonight with the martinis that she slammed down on an empty stomach. We won't take her anywhere and when her boyfriend gets here you can talk with him."

"Okay, but do NOT leave that table. I'm going to bring her some pasta. She needs to eat more than the appetizers if she hasn't eaten all day."

"Thank you."

"And I'm calling your office. But I won't call anyone else until after her boyfriend gets here."

"I understand. Thank you so much."

Melissa returned to the table and looked at Anthony. Bea was twirling her thumb drive on the table like a fidget spinner, stopping it intermittently to spin it again. It made a whirring sound that soothed her in her blurry state of mind.

"Look what I was able to find," Sandy said as she approached the table with a bowl of pappardelle covered with the meaty Bolognese gravy. "We DID have some Bolognese after all!"

"Yay!" Bea exclaimed, reaching for the bowl and a fork. "Bolognese!"

She wrapped one of the perfectly cooked noodles around the fork and stabbed at a piece of sausage, putting the impeccably prepared pasta into her mouth.

"OH. MY. GOD." she exclaimed, rolling her eyes back into her head. "This is heavenly." Bea savored the taste of the Bolognese in her mouth, swallowed and refilled her fork for more.

"So, tell me about your boyfriend," Sandy asked, not wanting to leave Bea alone with her tablemates.

"He's handsome and sweet and hikes and has a dog named Rufus and works with his mom at the animal clinic and . . ." Bea rambled as she continued to consume the pasta dish.

"Is his name Jaime? Are you dating Jaime Britton?"

"Yes! You know Jaime?" Bea asked excitedly, thrilled to meet someone that knew him.

"Yes, Jaime and I go way back. He's been coming here for years. I take my dogs to him for all of the shots and stuff. He's a great guy." Sandy was relieved that someone she knew and trusted was coming to take care of Bea. "How long have you been going out?"

"Maybe a month? He fell down a cliff and I washed off his chest."

"Well, okay then," Sandy laughed. "How's that Bolognese? Is it making you feel better?"

"Yes, it's so good and I was SO hungry. I thought I ordered another drink a while ago?"

"Oh, let's not worry about that right now. Besides, Jaime's on his way," Sandy turned to Anthony, "Should I get you the check?"

"Yes, please," replied Anthony, relieved that Sandy knew Jaime and was relaxing a bit over the situation. Sandy headed back into the kitchen as Anthony finished his Negroni.

Melissa looked outside as she caught movement from the corner of her eye. Vinnie was starting to get out of his chair as someone was walking through the door. Anthony and Bea had their backs toward the window and weren't able to see what was happening.

"Vinnie!" Melissa said quickly, getting up from her seat.

"Shit," said Anthony, looking over his shoulder as Vinnie was beginning to turn towards the door. He grabbed Bea and pulled her towards the kitchen – Melissa in tow.

"Bea?" Jaime said, walking in, the door closing behind him.

"Hi, honey!" she sang to Jaime while being tucked behind the wall in the galley. Jaime walked briskly to the back of the restaurant to join her.

"What the hell?" Sandy demanded, seeing the three customers standing beside her in the kitchen, Jaime joining them.

"Yeah, seriously, what in the hell is happening here?" Jaime chimed in.

"Just give us one minute – please. Otherwise, Bea may lose her job. Just one minute," Anthony explained, glancing around the wall to see Vinnie walking to the restrooms at the back of the restaurant, adjacent to the kitchen. He put his finger to his lips and mouthed, "shhh."

"Shhhhhhhh," hissed Bea obediently.

"Shhh," Melissa echoed, nodding her head in approval to Bea.

Sandy and Jaime looked at each other, exasperated with the situation. Finally, Sandy grabbed Bea by the arm and led her out the back door, the others following.

"Spill it," Sandy demanded of Anthony. "I'm done with this."

Chapter 13

"It's actually quite simple," Anthony started.

"I want to hear from her," Sandy said, pointing to Bea.

"But she's . . ." started Melissa.

"I want to hear this from Bea as well," Jaime interrupted.

Bea looked at Sandy and Jaime and asked, "What do you want to know?"

Jaime took Bea by the hand and asked, "Who are these two people and why are you here with them?"

"Oh, this is Mitch-Anthony and this is Jessica-Melissa," Bea replied. "They used to just be Mitch and Jessica when I met them on my business trip in Virginia, but now they're Anthony and Melissa."

"And why are they Anthony and Melissa now?" Jaime asked slowly.

"Because the other names were fake ones," Bea responded. "That way the mafia guys wouldn't know they were reporters from the Washington Post."

"What?" Jamie asked loudly, turning to Anthony. "What did you get her involved in?" he asked pointedly.

"Nothing," Anthony said, backing up with his hands up in front of him. "She was already employed by Medicroy when I met her in Virginia. I had taken a job as security personnel to get information for a story we're working on. Yes, there are mafia ties but just as an investment from what I can tell. Anytime there's as much money involved as there is with Gelinex and Medicroy, the mafia is going to be involved."

"Gelinex? The pharmaceutical company?" Jaime asked him.

"Yes, Medicroy and Gelinex are working together on CBD products. Medicroy is running conflicting studies – one to show that CBD is dangerous and should be scheduled for pharma use only, and the other to show the safety and efficacy of a cannabidiol-based drug that they've submitted for fast-track FDA approval."

"I didn't know!" Bea exclaimed, throwing her hands up to her face and crying into them, shaking her head fiercely. Too fiercely, in fact, as she fell over to one side and into Melissa, nearly taking her out in the process.

"Let me grab her a chair – but don't say a word. I don't want to miss any of this," demanded Sandy, disappearing into the kitchen and then back with a folding chair for Bea.

Sandy helped Bea into the chair. Bea was still crying, saying, "I didn't know" over and over again.

Jaime knelt by Bea's chair and said softly, "Let's not worry

about this right now. I just need to know what's happening.
There's a lot to take in, so if you could try to calm down and
stop crying, that would really be helpful."

Bea's crying escalated and she was now in the throws of full-on
sobbing. "But I didn't know! And I'm going to testify in front
of Congress against them and reveal everything and lose my
job!" she cried.

"What in the hell is she talking about?" Jaime demanded of
Anthony, turning away from the overly drunk and distraught
Bea.

"I really think we just need to take a breath here," Anthony
started.

"I swear to God . . . " started Jaime, staring Anthony down.

"Please," said Anthony. "I'll tell you everything. I've got
nothing to hide. But can we do it away from this?" he asked,
gesturing towards Bea who was being comforted by Melissa
and Sandy.

Jaime stared at Anthony for several seconds, nodded his head
and walked towards the kitchen and waved for Anthony to
follow him.

They walked back into the restaurant from the kitchen and came
face to face with Vinnie, who was headed back to his table from
the men's room.

"Mitch – what are you doing here?" Vinnie asked, looking at him and Jaime.

Anthony threw his arms up in the air and sighed in exasperation.

"He came to visit his brother and mother. Have a problem with that?" Jaime asked briskly, not wanting to out Anthony until he knew the entire story.

"No, no problem here," Vinnie replied defensively, moving past the men and towards the patio. "Just surprised, that's all."

"Grab the stuff from the table," Jaime instructed Anthony and went back through the kitchen and out the back door.

"You," said Jaime, pointing towards Melissa. "Take your car to the far end of the building and we'll meet you there with Bea."

"Don't go through the restaurant", cautioned Anthony. "I just ran into Vinnie in there. Jaime covered for me but he's not going to buy it if he sees you."

"Anthony," Jaime said, "pay Sandy and meet me at Melissa's car with all the stuff. I'm going to help Bea walk over there."

"Awww, man," Sandy whined. "I'm going to miss the good stuff. You have to fill me in later."

"Done," Jaime agreed. "Anthony, you'd better tip the hell out of her."

"That goes without saying," Anthony replied, pulling out his wallet.

Everyone met at Jaime's house after Domenic's to bring him up to speed. Jaime had stopped by Bea's to pick up Izzie on the way. Izzie was excited to see him and sat across from him on the front seat of his car with her front paws crossed elegantly in front of her.

"You sure are no Rufus," he said to her, laughing.

Jaime pulled up to his place about five minutes later. Anthony, Melissa and Bea had already arrived and had gone into the house where Bea was gleefully received by Rufus. She had introduced him to the others and he followed them in and sat at Bea's feet until Jaime arrived.

Jaime walked in and gently lowered Izzie to the floor with one hand while holding an excited, butt-wiggling Rufus at bay with the other. Izzie went immediately to the overstuffed chair by the window and glared at Anthony who was the current occupant. Rufus followed closely behind, tail wagging fiercely.

"That's her chair," Jaime informed Anthony, who immediately got up and relinquished the seat to Izzie. A guest in Jaime's house, he wasn't going to ask any questions – especially since Jaime didn't blow his cover with Vinnie. There was still some work to be done on the exposé he and Melissa were working on, and he needed a couple more weeks working for "the boys" to wrap it up.

Jaime walked over to Bea who was sitting on the couch and sat beside her. "How are you feeling?" he asked her, trying to gauge the Purple Haze effect level.

"I'm okay," she replied. "I'm just a little drunk right now but I'm okay. It's been an interesting day."

"Yes, I can see that," Jaime laughed. Turning to the others, "I can throw some hamburgers on if anyone's hungry. It's not as good as Domenic's but you don't have to dodge any bosses and fake your identity here."

"That would be great," Anthony chuckled. "Can I give you a hand?"

"Sure, I'll meet you out back."

Jaime went into the kitchen and Melissa took his place on the couch next to Bea.

"Anthony said that you want to work with us on the story. Is that right?"

"Yes, I want to expose those assholes. I can't believe they put me in this position. But right now, I really gotta pee."

Bea stood up and steadied herself. She kicked off her shoes and walked towards the bathroom, using the walls as support along the way.

Melissa joined Anthony on the back porch and asked, "Do you think Vinnie bought Jaime's story?"

"He's surprisingly good at lying," Anthony replied. "I think he bought it, but I'm going to stop in at Medicroy on Monday and say 'Hi' to Sarcos since I'm 'in town visiting family' just to make sure."

"Good idea. With Bea's help, this is going to be an amazing story. We're going to need to spread this over several articles so we can go in depth into it. We may need to get the video guys involved and turn this into a feature."

"I'll text them and get it set up. If Bea's up to it, let's get some time with her this weekend and go through her data to get that nailed down. Man, this has been a wild one, huh?"

"Definitely, but worth it. Who knows, we may be able to pull a Pulitzer for it if we do it right. At the very least, we'll get national press on it. You can't get a hotter topic than cannabis mixed with greed, dirty politicians and a cover up."

"Yeah, about all that," Jaime started, walking onto the patio with a tray of food for the grill, "let's pick up where we left off at Domenic's."

Anthony filled Jaime in on who the two of them were, the Virginia trip, the article they were working on and how Bea fits into the picture, while Jaime prepped the patties and got them on the grill. Melissa told him everything she knew about the conflicting studies that they were running and Medicroy's upcoming presentation to the Ways and Means Committee, Bea's NDA, NORML's take on that and their offer to defend her should it become necessary, and their request for her to testify with them directly after Sarcos' testimony.

"So, she really had no idea then, did she?" Jaime asked.

"No, there's no way she knew what was happening," Anthony confirmed. "They were using her to complete the study, and by putting her name on it she would be tagged as anti-cannabis and would pretty much be stuck in that lane moving forward. The cannabis industry would blackball her for sure, and Medicroy would use that to keep her in her job long-term. She'd pretty much be stuck there because her integrity would be questioned by the scientific community at large. She'd never work as a scientist again outside of Medicroy or Gelinex."

"Damn. But NORML's going to support her?"

"100 percent. And with her revealing the findings that she told us about tonight on the oil from Chinese study, she will have the support of the entire industry. What they're doing would be considered criminal by most people's standards. At the very least, it's unethical."

"Fucking Medicroy. God, I can't wait to out them," Jaime growled.

"Let's get all of our ducks in a row first," Melissa countered.

"If we do this the right way, we can bury them. But we need to have everything verified. We need test results, documentation, statements from people involved – all of that – to make sure there are no holes in the story in case they want to take legal action against any of us. We're planning to release the first part of the story online directly following the testimony to Congress and an expanded version in the Post the next morning as the beginning of a series."

"I just don't want our town to be blindsided by this and made out to be oblivious to what's happening in our own backyard," Jaime asserted.

"You've lived your entire life here, have been involved in studies with CBD at CSU, and didn't even know who Medicroy was, let alone what they were up to." Anthony explained. "They are really good at flying under the radar, all the way down to their filings with the state. Nothing indicates that they're even a lab or that the lab has any certifications, let alone any CLIA certificates. They're using Gelinex's accreditations to run the studies, but they're putting it in Medicroy's name. That's some shady shit there and it'll be brought up in the article. We're not bringing the town into this. It's about Bill Sarcos, Vinnie Zabini and Congressman Jeffries – not about Fort Collins. This could have happened anywhere."

"I just can't believe that Bea got caught up in all of this. Speaking of which, I should go check on her. You guys can start eating. There are beers in the fridge."

Jaime returned to the house and made his way to the back of the house where Bea was headed earlier. As he walked down the hall, he heard noise coming from his bedroom which he was able to identify as snoring the closer he came to it. But not just regular snoring – a cacophony of snoring. Entering his bedroom, he found Bea, Rufus and Izzie all asleep on the bed, their snores battling each other in an invisible arena for top billing.

Letting "sleeping dogs lie," he returned to the patio to convene with his guests.

"Is she okay?" asked Melissa.

"She's sleeping it off in my bed with the dogs. How much did she drink?"

"She only had two martinis," Anthony explained. "But she downed them both in less than 5 minutes and hadn't eaten all day."

"Ohhhhhhhhh, yeah that'll do it. Besides that, she's really not that much of a drinker from what I know of her." Jaime replied. "She's not going to be much help tonight."

"She gave me her notebook and the thumb drive with the data on it. We could go through that, but I'm not a scientist so it's not going to make much sense to me."

"Let me take a look at it," Jamie offered. He took the notebook and reviewed the contents while he and his guests ate their burgers, occasionally making notes on a pad that he grabbed from a drawer below the pizza oven. He was engrossed in the data, occasionally blurting out a "holy shit" and "what the hell" when he found something overtly offensive, followed by vigorous bouts of writing and head shaking.

After about an hour of reading, eating and drinking, he finally closed the notebook and stated, "We need a plan."

Chapter 14

Jaime lit the citronella torches that surrounded the patio while Anthony worked on starting a fire in the fire pit. Melissa had already cleared the plates and brought the tray and leftovers into the kitchen when sleeping "Bea-ty" arrived on the patio.

"Hey there," Jaime said, welcoming Bea to the land of the conscious and relatively sober. "Did you have a nice nap?" he asked, kissing her on the cheek.

"Yes, thank you. What did I miss?"

"Oh, not much. Just a review of your findings on the study, a suggested outline for your counter-presentation at the Ways and Means Committee with NORML and a list of what we need you to sneak out of Medicroy Monday morning."

Bea stood there, not moving for a moment, staring at Jaime and the two reporters. She turned around and started to walk back inside.

"Hold on. It's going to be okay," Jaime laughed, going after her.

"This is just too much for me to handle right now. I'm not sober enough for all of this."

"I understand. We'll go over it all tomorrow morning. For

now, all you need to know is that it's going to be okay and that we're behind you. I'm behind you. And I'm going to help you."

Bea buried her face in Jaime's chest and started crying, "I didn't know! I really didn't know! And then I met you and fell in love and didn't know how to tell you and didn't want you to think that I was involved in all this and then Mitch and Jessica turned out to be Anthony and Melissa and . . ."

"It's okay, it's okay," Jaime stroked Bea's hair. "You don't have to worry about that anymore. They explained everything – well not about the falling in love, but . . ."

Bea quickly stood up and took a step back, covered her mouth with her hand, eyes big as saucers, horrified that she let that little piece of information slip.

"And you don't have to worry about that either. The feeling is mutual."

Jaime held his arms out for her to fold herself into and he closed them around her protectively, kissing her on the top of her head.

Anthony and Melissa looked at each other, gathered their belongings and walked towards the side of the house. Anthony signaled to Jaime that they were leaving, and took the flagstone path to the front of the house, leaving Bea and Jaime to themselves.

"Are you hungry?" Jaime asked Bea, her face still burrowed in his chest.

"No," she said, muffled, shaking her head back and forth.

"Thirsty?"

"No," muffled and shaking her head again.

"Want to sit out here and enjoy the fire for a while?"

"That would be nice." Bea untucked herself from Jaime slowly and peered towards the fire pit.

Jaime took her hand and led her over to the double chaise. She lowered herself onto the chaise and leaned back onto the reclined cushions while Jaime grabbed a large blanket from the outdoor chest under the window. He joined her on the chaise, covering them both with the blanket and leaned back, putting his arm out for her to come closer to him. She placed her head on his shoulder as he wrapped his arm around her and kissed her head.

The fire danced and crackled for the better part of an hour before either of them moved. They had been mesmerized by the flames and comforted by the soft breeze and the warmth of the blanket on the cloudless, chilly night. Rufus and Izzie had long retired to the house and were asleep on the couch, snoring.

"Are you disappointed in me?" Bea finally asked, afraid to hear the answer.

"For what?"

"For getting involved in this whole mess at Medicroy."

"No," Jaime held her closer. "You didn't know what was happening and they put you in a bad spot pretty quickly. You were just in the wrong place at the wrong time. Now, if you're talking about drinking two Purple Haze martinis at Domenic's in less than five minutes, I'm more impressed than disappointed."

"Yeah, that was a bit much."

"It sounds like it was warranted. But when I take you there next time, let's spread them out a bit more, okay?"

"Okay. They really were good. Do you know how to make those?"

"No, and I'm not going to learn. I think I'd have a booze hound on my hand if I did. Let's just leave those as a special treat for when we go to Domenic's. Agreed?"

"Agreed. That and the Bolognese."

"Yes, that and the Bolognese."

Anthony and Melissa had rejoined Jaime and Bea - who was

recovering from a slight hangover with the help of a couple droppers of CBD - the following morning. The three of them began the weekend preparing her notes, fine tuning her presentation and laying out the plan, step by step, leaving nothing to chance. Melissa worked on reorganizing the article with the new information and Anthony focused on scheduling the video crew and cluing them in on what was going to go down at the hearing. He knew what he wanted and there was only going to be one opportunity to get it, so he was leaving nothing to chance.

Bea was already at her desk Monday morning when she heard "Mitch" come in. He sauntered down the hallway and knocked on the open door going into Sarcos' office.

"Hey, boss man," Anthony offered. "I'm in town visiting family and thought I'd stop in and see the place."

"Vinnie said he saw you at Domenic's Friday night," Bill responded. "I didn't realize you had family here."

"Yeah, my brother and mother moved here a couple years back. I hadn't had the chance to visit, but my mom's not doing well so I thought I'd better come and spend a little time with her."

"Sorry to hear that. Come on in. When are you heading back?"

"Wednesday. I need to get back to headquarters before the testimony to make sure everything is locked down and secure. Even though the testimony is coming from Medicroy, I don't want any leaks coming out of Gelinex, so I'm going to be checking everyone as they leave the office next Thursday to make sure nothing goes home with them before Friday's testimony."

"I never thought about that."

"That's why you guys hired me. I can set up someone here to do the same if you want."

"Thanks, but I think we're good here. The only ones that know anything are me and Bea, and I don't have to worry about either of us."

"True, you don't have to deal with the amount of staff that we have at the lab. It's nice to be able to keep it small that way."

"You got that right," a voice from behind him declared. Anthony turned around to see Vinnie standing behind him with the third man that he didn't recognize from their meeting at Domenic's Friday evening.

"Mitch, how long you here for?" Vinnie asked Anthony. "There are a couple things I could use a little help with if you have some extra time."

"Sure thing," Anthony replied. "I'm here until Wednesday, but I have some time here and there. What 'cha need?"

"It's more what he needs," Vinnie said, referring to the man standing next to him. "This is Chad Ellis – he's helping Billy prepare for the presentation. It's too important to leave to chance, so we're doing a few trial runs."

Anthony held his hand out and shook Chad's hand. Chad looked like he came straight off a modeling job, perfectly dressed, not a hair out of place and shoes that were shined to the point of needing sunglasses because of their glare.

"I could use some people to make up a panel," Chad explained, in a deep, confident voice. "I know that Bill has a lot of experience presenting, but the panel will be asking some pointed questions – questions that we just happen to have ahead of time – and we want him to practice his responses in an organic way so he'll be ready for them."

"So, you need me to round up some people to serve as the panel?" asked Anthony.

"Precisely. And although the committee will be throwing him softballs, I'd like the panel to be a little harsher on him just in case."

"Bring it on," quipped Bill from his desk. "The bitchier the better. Go get me some middle-aged housewives to be on the panel. And some wound-up liberals from Boulder while you're at it. Can't get much worse than that!"

Bill and his two cohorts laughed and added some additional suggestions along the same vein while Anthony bit his tongue in anticipation of the laugh ultimately being on them Friday.

"I'm on it!" agreed Anthony.

"Get me six to eight angry liberals. We'll pay them $200 each for the day. Set it up for tomorrow at the Elizabeth Hotel. We've already reserved the space for it," Vinnie instructed. "We'll even throw in lunch."

"Consider it done," Anthony said, turning to leave.

"Maybe put your brother on the panel - he seemed a little tightly wound Friday," Vinnie suggested.

"Maybe I will," Anthony replied and headed out the door, making eye contact with Bea across the hall. She nodded to him from behind her desk and he mouthed "I'll text you," and left.

The following day, Bea joined Sarcos, Vinnie, Chad and Anthony at the Elizabeth Hotel where the panel had been formed, seated behind tables arranged similarly to how the members would be seated at the hearing. An empty table was across from them where Bill and Chad took their positions. Vinnie, Bea and Anthony sat in chairs at the back of the room where Bea and Anthony barely exchanged words and didn't acknowledge Jaime, who was going over the questions that he had been given by Chad for the mock testimony. Bea took out her notebook and started making notes for both Sarcos' testimony and her own that would be following it.

The mock testimony started with Sarcos giving his presentation to the mock committee. Bea could see Jaime taking notes at certain points and hoped that he would not do anything that might blow his cover or jeopardize the plan. The longer Sarcos spoke, the more irritated Jaime seemed to get and the more he would write. She'd never seen this side of him and wasn't sure what might come next.

Fortunately, she didn't have to wait long to find out as the presentation ended and Jaime was the first up to ask questions. He was given his five minutes to question Bill. He read the first question that had been prepared by Chad, "Can you explain to us what cannabinoids are and how they work in your body?"

Sarcos rattled off his pat answer, pleased with the softball that had been tossed to him and how he was able to hit it out of the park.

Then Jaime asked his second question – one that hadn't been prepared by Chad, "Why would you suggest that a phytocannabinoid would be any more dangerous than an equivalent endocannbinoid that is produced naturally by the body?"

Sarcos paused, startled at the question that he had not been expecting.

"Good! Good!" Chad said to Jaime. "I like the energy. I didn't expect that, but that's okay. We'll need to practice things like that in case someone throws us a curveball, but let's stick to the prepared questions for now and we'll ease into the non-scripted after lunch."

"Let's go to the next panel member. Karen, how about you?" Chad directed.

Jaime shot a quick glance at Bea, who was sitting by Anthony in the back of the room, and then focused again on Sarcos, waiting for his chance to question him again.

"Damn, he's a little bulldog," Vinnie whispered to Anthony, leaning over Bea. "Must have been a barrel of laughs growing up with that one."

"You have no idea," Anthony replied – who truly had no idea since they had only met days before.

Chapter 15

Wednesday came and went with Anthony catching a flight back to Jersey and Chad and Sarcos fine-tuning the presentation and responses to the questions that had been provided.

Bea quietly worked on her own presentation, getting additional data from Adam, the Lab Rat, who she had since filled in on what Medicroy and Gelinex were doing and their plan to expose it. After work, she spent time going over the more complex inner-workings of the endocannabinoid system with Jaime – and some of his own personal complex inner-workings as well.

Thursday morning, Sarcos and Chad took the corporate jet to Jersey to finish preparing, leaving Bea at the office to tie up loose ends, make any changes to the presentation that had been noted and get them to the committee by the end of the day so they could be reviewed before the testimony the next afternoon.

Bea was nose-deep in her notes, going over every last bit of data to make sure she hadn't missed anything when she heard a knock on her door.

"Hey, Adam," Bea said, welcoming him. "What's up?"

"I just wanted to wish you good luck for tomorrow. I know it's gonna be hard to do what you have to do, but you're doing it for the right reason and I respect the hell out of you for that," Adam confessed. "I'm pretty sure they're going to have changed the locks to the office by the time you get back. Do you have anything lined up work-wise?"

"No, I can't really do anything until after it all goes down tomorrow. It's too risky, and what am I going to say? That I'm testifying against a study that I co-wrote for an employer who's back-dealing with a pharma company and basically lying to the FDA? I'm going to have to wait until it all comes out in the Post and cross my fingers that I find something soon. I have a little money saved up and my credit cards are paid down, so that will buy me a month or two, but that's about it."

"If there's anything that I can do, just let me know."

"You know, this may close the entire lab down. Are YOU going to be okay?"

"Me? Yeah, no worries there. I'll be fine."

"No, seriously. You might lose your job because of this. If you need any help, you can stay at my place. I have an extra bedroom and you can even have your own bathroom if you need a place to stay while you look for another job. I hate that you might be unemployed because of this."

Adam smiled and chuckled, realizing that Bea had no idea who he was, other than a Lab Rat at Medicroy.

"Bea, you have nothing to worry about when it comes to me. I'm a Singerson. My grandfather founded the largest manufacturing company in the state. I didn't take this job for the money, I took it to learn about the industry. I just didn't realize that I was learning about it from a piece of shit like Sarcos. I was serious when I said if there's anything I can do to let me know. I've learned more from you than I could have ever learned from anyone else. Including integrity. If you need ANYTHING, let me know."

Bea was dumbfounded at the revelation. In all of her interactions with Adam, she never really thought of his life outside of the walls of the lab – his family or friends – just that he was a smart, dedicated and gifted young man with a thirst for knowledge.

"This has been a VERY strange month," she finally said, just shaking her head.

"I hear you. But I mean what I said. You have my number. Let's get together when you get back in town and talk. I'll be watching C-SPAN tomorrow. Can't wait to see you lay it to the boss man!"

"Yeah, lay it to the boss man," Bea said nervously as Adam went back to the lab.

When Bea arrived home, she saw Jaime's Jeep in her driveway. Her heart skipped a beat as she really needed a boost after all of the planning and preparing they had been doing that week - all of which would end up leading to the demise of her job and possibly her career.

She parked alongside his car and entered through the front door to see Jaime giving Izzie her CBD.

"Is everything okay?" she asked, wondering about the surprise visit.

"Everything's fine," he said, walking towards her to give her a kiss. "I just wanted to spend some time with you tonight, so I thought we could all go out for a picnic dinner and wanted to give Izzie her CBD before we went."

"That's so sweet. Let me change into something more comfortable and then we can go."

"I'll load up the Jeep and wait for you out front." Jaime grabbed the basket of food, a bottle of wine and the dogs.

Bea went to her room and threw on some jeans and a t-shirt for the evening, grabbing a hoodie off the dresser on the way out in case it got chilly. As she headed to the front door, the house phone rang. It startled her as she'd never heard it ring before because she had never given that number to anyone. The only reason she even had it was because it was free with the bundled internet and cable promo.

She picked up that phone and answered, "Hello?"

"Don't do it. You'll regret it," the voice on the phone said and hung up.

Bea stood there, alone, shocked and truly afraid for the first time since this all started. Sure, she had been on guard at times, especially in Virginia, and had been worried multiple times over the last several months with the layer upon layers of deceit being revealed. She never considered that someone might harm her – that it was anything other than just setting the record straight and telling the truth. But that naivete was now stripped away as she stood there with a phone in her hand and the sound of a dial tone emanating from it. She had been threatened and the voice was ringing in her ears. It all seemed different now – much, much different.

Bea sat on her couch, clad in her blue jeans and t-shirt, clutching her hoodie. She stared straight ahead, the threat from the caller running through her mind over and over again. Several minutes had passed when Jaime came in to check on her.

"Couldn't find anything to wear?" he joked, walking into the living room. "Hey, what's up?" he asked, seeing her sitting there, staring into space like a zombie. "What's happening?"

"I got a call," was all she could get out. "I got a call."

"What call?"

"I got a call on the phone," Bea pointed to the house phone on the kitchen counter, tearing up.

"Is everyone okay? Did something happen to your mom?"

"He threatened me. He said, 'Don't do it- you'll regret it' and hung up. They know." Tears streamed down her face in fear.

Jaime jumped up and grabbed the phone, looking for the caller ID.

"Amateur," Jaime mumbled, pulled out his cell phone out and placed a call.

"I have a number, find him," he simply said, giving the person on the other end of the call the phone number and then hanging up.

Jaime walked over to the couch and sat by Bea. "I won't let anything happen to you. You'll be fine, nobody can hurt you. I'm here and won't let anything happen to you."

"But you won't be there tomorrow," she said, looking into his eyes. "And what about the next day? And the day after that? What about my family? And Izzie? Are you going to be with them too to protect them? And you don't even know who it is? How can you protect me if you don't even know who it is?" Tears ran down Bea's cheeks as she continued to hold on to her hoodie like a security blanket.

"Bea, it's just someone trying to scare you. If it was a real threat, they would have been smart enough to block their number. Who has this number?"

"Nobody. I don't even know the number. It's on my paperwork somewhere, but I've never used it. The cable company just said I had to set it up and activate it to get the discount. That's the only reason I even have it." Bea headed towards the kitchen and started rummaging through a drawer.

Just then Jaime's cell phone rang. He answered it without saying a word, listening to the voice on the other end. "Get eyes on him," Jaime said quietly and hung up.

Jaime stood up and headed towards the kitchen, "Let me get Rufus and Izzie out of the car and bring the basket back in. How about we have the picnic right here? Would that be better? I stopped by Trader Joe's and got your favorite popcorn and pickles," he cooed, coercing an "almost smile" from her. "I'll move the table and spread the blanket on the floor and we'll have dinner right here. I'll even put Izzie and Rufus out back with treats so they don't fight us for the food. Come on, what do you say? I won't let you leave my sight."

"Okay, I'm just too freaked out right now to go anywhere."

"I hear you. It's completely understandable. I totally get why you're feeling that way. Let me just get the dogs and the basket and I'll be right back. Do you want to watch me from the door?"

"Yeah, I don't want to be alone, even if it's just for a minute. I'm afraid the phone's going to ring again," she said, truly frightened.

"Trust me. It's not going to ring again."

The next morning, Bea woke up in Jaime's arms with Rufus on the other side of her and Izzie on her thigh.

"Well, you can't get more protected than this," she thought to herself, the shock from the call last night lessening a bit and a small pinch of Jaime's voice of reason finding its way through a crack in the wall she had thrown up. "I'm not going to ignore it, but I'm not going to change my plans. I'll just have to keep my eyes and ears open," she decided. "Besides, I'll have Anthony there with me and he's not going to let anything happen to me."

Jaime had called Anthony the evening before and caught him up on what had happened. Anthony, having served in the Marines, assured Jaime that he would be at her side the entire time and would have backup with him as well. He would be waiting for her at the airport to bring her to the hearing and wouldn't leave her side.

Anthony had asked Jaime if he had any leads on who it could have been and Jaime told him not to worry about it. He had some friends looking into it for him and left it at that.

Rufus rolled over onto his back and let out a ridiculously long and smelly fart that smelled like it had been released from the depths of hell. Bea started struggling to be released from under the covers and Jaime sprang out of bed to open a window.

"GOOD GOD!" Jaime exclaimed. "That's VILE!"

Rufus lay there on his back, tail wagging, while even Izzie jumped off the bed, fleeing for cleaner air.

"No more treats for you," Jaime threatened. "Not if that's the thanks I get."

"What was in those treats? Old eggs and chicken livers?" Bea asked through a t-shirt that she had covered her face with. She ran to the bathroom and came back with a can of air freshener, blasting the room as if she were clearing out demons during an exorcism. "Let's hope that this isn't an omen for how the day is going to go."

"Well, if it is, then I have faith you will handle it. We'll just have to slip a can of air freshener into your bag," Jaime kissed her through the t-shirt.

Bea laughed and removed the t-shirt so they could have a proper kiss as Rufus jumped off the bed and headed towards the living room.

"How are you feeling today?" Jaime asked.

"I'm better. Still a little freaked out, but better. Thank you for staying last night. And Rufus. Truthfully, if you could train Rufus to fart like that on demand, he could be a real lifesaver for me."

"True, but you'd get caught in the crossfire and I couldn't risk that," Jaime kissed her again.

Bea dropped the air freshener on the floor and pulled Jaime back into bed on top of her. There would be no need for Rufus' protection right now.

Chapter 16

Jaime took Bea to the airport and walked her to the CLEAR security entrance. She caught the train to Gate C and boarded the Southwestern 7am flight to DC. The flight would arrive in time to get her to the hearing's afternoon session where Sarcos would be testifying, then followed by NORML.

Bea had a high boarding number and knew that she would be stuck in a middle seat, but hoped that she would at least be able to get some time to review her notes without being elbowed the entire time. As she followed the line of people into the plane's cabin, a gentleman caught her attention. He had chatted with her in the terminal for a moment before the first boarding group of "status" flyers had been called at which time he and his friend boarded. He waved her over to the row that he and his friend were sitting in, got up and took the middle seat, offering her the aisle.

"Are you sure?" she asked.

"Definitely," he replied, generously. "I wouldn't ask you to sit next to Eric. He's an old sod," he cracked, his British accent making the insult sound like a line from a Monty Python movie.

"Thank you so much!" she gushed, thrilled to have a little extra room for the flight. She quickly got settled and pulled out her notes to review for the umpteenth time. There wasn't anything that she didn't know in the notes like the back of her hand, but seeing Sarcos startled at the mock testimony made her worry that she might freeze as well, and she couldn't afford to do that.

The flight was uneventful. She shared some conversation with her aisle mates, explaining the science of cannabinoids and the basics of the endocannabinoid system. Eric and Graham, the gentleman who offered her his seat, asked thoughtful questions and she took her time answering them with specific examples when possible. They seemed genuinely interested in the subject and she enjoyed passing the time with them talking about the science – the facts – surrounding the cannabinoids.

They walked with her through the terminal, picking her brain the entire time about minor cannabinoids and terpenes and receptors, soaking up all the knowledge that Bea offered. They promised that they would keep themselves up to date on the FDA's stance on the promising herb. As they made their way towards baggage claim, Bea spotted Anthony and introduced the gentlemen to him. He shook their hands as they explained how she had just given them a lesson on the cannabis plant and everything surrounding it and they were going to go find some CBD "straight away" and try it.

Bea laughed and gave them each a hug before leaving with Anthony, even more staunch in her decision to speak up against Medicroy that afternoon. THEY were the reason that she was doing this. Those gentlemen and the rest of the people that can benefit from CBD – away from the unwarranted clutches and high cost of big pharma. They were the "why" of what she was doing - especially Eric, as he had been suffering from restless leg syndrome. Bea had given him specific articles to read in addition to a study done by a pharmaceutical company that showed up to 50 percent of participants had benefitted from their patented cannabis-based drug. Similar results had been found by simply taking CBD – a much more natural choice without any side effects, unlike the pharma drug that had been used in the study.

Bea practically floated through the airport terminal and to the waiting car. Anthony joined her in the back, the driver whisking them away to Capitol Hill, as she regaled him with pieces of the conversation that they had shared on the flight. Anthony offered her an avocado, egg salad and sprouts sandwich on wheat (Melissa's recommendation) along with a LIFEWTR to wash it down with, as there would be no time to stop for lunch before getting to the capitol, and it was going to be a long afternoon.

Anthony told Bea that Melissa would be there for her testimony but would be in the listening room for Sarcos' part, so as not to draw attention as Vinnie would be there. Sarcos, Vinnie and Chad had been there all day, watching and listening to testimony and gauging the interest of the members. They were grabbing lunch and would meet them there, but Anthony would not leave her side – even if it meant blowing his cover. He would not leave her side.

Sarcos gave his testimony, Congressman Jeffries and his cronies lobbing softballs at him. Bea sat in the chairs behind him with Vinnie Zambini, Steve Lyons, and Chad Ellis on one side of her and Anthony on her other side.

The committee had submitted their questions to the chair who reviewed them and had, in turn, covertly provided them to Congressman Jeffries for him to pass along to his buddy to prepare with. They had artfully prepared answers to even the toughest questions, phrasing them in a way to cast doubt on the safety of cannabinoids. But what they had not prepared for was what came after the first question in their allotted five minutes: the follow-up questions. And there were a handful of representatives that sounded as if they were channeling Jaime, down to the tone of his voice, including the Representative from Colorado.

"Do you have any evidence of overdose from cannabidiol?" asked Colorado's Representative Calhoun.

"The science is not conclusive on that matter," Sarcos replied.

"It's not conclusive or it's not giving you the results that support your agenda? How do you substantiate any danger from the use of cannabidiol?"

"Our study clearly shows that the subjects' health deteriorated after using cannabidiol."

"Your study shows that the subjects' health deteriorated after using your specific tincture," the representative clarified. "It does not show that the adverse effects came from cannabidiol alone. Perhaps your tincture was compromised. Do you have a certificate of analysis on the specific tincture you used?"

"Yes, of course," Sarcos directed him to the page in his presentation where he had inserted the COA for the Colorado oil in the place of the Chinese oil.

"You understand that you are under oath?"

"Yes," Sarcos replied, startled at the implication.

"And you're stating that this COA is the COA for the oil that you provided to the participants in the study?"

"Yes," Sarcos tried to sound confident.

"No more questions. I yield the balance of my time."

Questioning continued for another 20 minutes or so before Sarcos' testimony was over. He left the table and sat in the empty seat beside Anthony.

"The committee calls Derek Sanders, special counsel to NORML," the committee Chairman stated.

Chad turned to Bea, "Hold my beer," he said – although he had no beer - stood up and approached the table.

"I'm Dr. Derek Sanders," he stated before being sworn in.

There was not a jaw that was not agape in the row of seats that

Bea occupied. Bea's stomach and head were fighting for the "Most Active in Case of Emergency" award, while Vinnie, Sarcos and Steve Lyons started talking over each other - getting a warning from the committee Chairman to not speak while in his chambers.

Just then, Melissa walked in and took Chad/Derek's seat.

"Didn't see that coming!" she whispered to Bea. "NORML said they had a plant, but I didn't know it was him!"

Vinnie looked at Jessica/Melissa and told Steve to switch seats with him.

"Jessica, what are you doing here?" he whispered to Melissa.

"Watching the show," she whispered back, handing him her business card from the Post. "And the name's Melissa."

Vinnie took the business card and read it. "What the hell?" he blurted.

"There will be order," declared the Chairman. "If you have matters that need to be taken care of, take it outside. If it happens again, you will be removed."

Vinnie stood, up grabbed Melissa by the arm and tried to pull her out of her seat. Anthony immediately stood up, grabbed Vinnie's arm and twisted it behind his back while putting his other hand on the back of Vinnie's neck.

"She's with the fucking Post," he yelled to Sarcos as security rushed over to remove him from the room. "Sarcos, she's with the Washington Post. We've been set up," he exclaimed as he was being dragged down the aisle.

"You can't set someone up that devised the plan in the first place," Derek called after him.

"Ma'am, can you please come with us so we can clarify a few things," a guard asked Melissa.

"Of course," Melissa offered, leaving with the guard.

Steve Lyons moved over to the empty seat next to Bea, removing his jacket and laying it over his lap.

"Dr. Sanders, please continue," the Chairman requested.

"As I was saying, I am here on the behalf of NORML, the National Organization for the Reform of Marijuana Laws. While the public may not realize this, up until the Farm Bill of 2018 passed, cannabidiol was included in the federal definition of marijuana and was treated as a schedule 1 drug. Because of this, the ability to do studies on CBD was severely stifled for organizations other than pharmaceutical companies. And, until recently, the pharmaceutical companies did not release any of these studies. Now that the restrictions have been removed and studies are being released every week showing cannabidiol's efficacy, pharmaceutical companies are releasing their own studies to try to instill fear into the public around CBD and secure scheduling to where they are the only sector that can have access to it."

Just then, the doors to the chambers opened and five uniformed officers, led by a gentleman in a dark suit, approached the row of seats that Medicroy was occupying.

"Steve Lyons, please come with us," stated the gentleman in the dark suit.

Steve quickly put one arm behind Bea and grabbed her neck. With his other hand, he grabbed a syringe from under his jacket and held it to Bea's throat.

"Yeah, I don't think so," Steve growled, the needle pushing up against the skin on Bea's neck.

Bea's body was as stiff as a board, afraid to even move, she held her breath, thinking it might be her last. How had it come to this? What kind of people would go to this extent for greed? "It's a plant, for God's sake," she thought to herself. "I'm going to die because some greedy bastard doesn't want to let people have access to a freaking herb."

Steve let go of her neck and grabbed her by the hair, yanking her head back to expose more of her neck. "There's no way I'm going to jail over this," he said, applying more pressure with the syringe to her neck, nearly piercing the skin. "I've worked too hard on this project to . . ." THUMP.

Lyons collapsed into Bea's lap and rolled onto the floor, blood slowly trickling onto the floor from where he had been hit in the back of his head.

"God, he's a prick," the man seated behind Bea muttered, slinging a small nylon sack with what appeared to have an 8-ball in it. He stood up and looked at the gentleman in the dark suit and asked, "You ready for him, Jerry?"

"Yes, we'll take it from here," he replied.

The police entered the row and secured Lyons in cuffs before they held smelling salts under his nose to bring him around. He came to and immediately tried to wrestle his hands from the cuffs.

"Hey," yelled the man with the 8-ball. "Don't push your luck."

Steve made eye contact with the man and quickly silenced himself, recognizing the mysterious figure looking down at him. As the officers lifted him off the ground, he never lost eye contact with the man that had knocked him out. He looked at him sheepishly, almost apologetically, and did not utter a word as he left with the officers and the man in the black suit.

The chairman slammed the gavel down with anger, "I. WILL. HAVE. ORDER!" he yelled. He ordered the chambers cleared other than Dr. Derek Sanders. Bea sat motionless, unable to coerce her body to move.

Sarcos, typically the brightest person in the room, had no idea what was going on. "Vinnie's girlfriend is a reporter? Lyons attacked Bea? Chad is special counsel for NORML? What in the hell is going on?" he asked no one in particular as he and the others made their way to the doors.

"Do you need assistance, young lady?" the Chairman asked. "You can take your time, but we will need you to leave as well. Just take the time you need, and we can get you some assistance if you need it."

"Actually," Derek interjected, "she'll be testifying with me for NORML."

"WHAT?!" Sarcos screamed from the back of the room, pushing his way back towards Bea. "I'll fucking bury you!" he yelled.

Anthony grabbed him, spun him around and looked him in the eye. "I've been looking for a reason to deck you for weeks now. Give me a reason," he said with grit in his voice. "Give me a reason!"

"Security, clear the room - everyone but Sanders and the young lady. Everyone – OUT," demanded the Chairman.

Congressman Jeffries sat quietly, trying to make himself look small in the chair. When Sarcos pointed to him and said, "Do something, Jeffries," he quickly left the chambers through the back door with his staff in tow. None of his cronies even looked at him. United they stand, divided they fall. And Jeffries had just fallen, hard and alone.

Derek and Bea spent the next four hours giving testimony to the Chairman and the members of the committee. The ones who had teamed with Jeffries earlier were now more open to listen to the science and asked constructive questions as a way to distance themselves from both him and Gelinex. And it would be easier for those politicians to explain away the millions of dollars in contributions they received from the company if they now threw their support behind legislation which promoted easier access to CBD and earmarked money for CBD research.

When their testimony ended, Derek and Bea gathered their belongings and walked towards the door in the back of the room to leave the chambers. They were met by a member of security.

"Tell Jaime 'hey' for me," the gentleman said, giving Bea his card. "It was an honor to do this for him after all he did for me. I'll always be in his debt."

Bea looked at him, wondering what he could possibly be talking about. He led them to a side door instead, and escorted them through the back halls into a waiting car that whisked them off to the small airport that Bea had last visited on the Gelinex jet.

This time a much larger jet was waiting for both her and Derek. And inside the jet waited a casually dressed gentleman with a smile on his face.

"I'm so glad to finally meet you," he said, shaking Bea's hand.

"I've heard such great things about you."

Bea looked at him, puzzled at who the gentleman was. A door opened at the back of the jet and things became abundantly clear.

"I told you I'd be watching on CSPAN," Adam declared. "Dad thought you might need a lift home."

Chapter 17

Bea spent the next day wavering between exhilaration and fear for the future. Between Twitter, LinkedIn, Snapchat and Instagram, #CBDBea was trending everywhere. She was deluged with calls and emails from reporters, and texts from friends and family who saw her on the news. Bea had little time to think about what had transpired the day before, due to the whirlwind of publicity she now found herself in.

Jaime had met her at the private airport in Loveland when she arrived the night before and brought her back to his house before the late night news and shows had begun. She was surprised to see that The 11th Hour with Brian Williams had used a clip from her testimony in a segment on CBD, and had convened a panel including NORML's Executive Director, a hemp-friendly senator and an industry leader as panelists to discuss all things cannabis. By the next morning she had received invitations from The Late Show with Stephen Colbert, The Today Show and also from the ladies at The View to discuss the safety and benefits of CBD on their shows.

She was glad to have gotten a text from Adam Singerson that morning, and asked him if he could come over and help her wade through the social media and email submissions that were coming through. He had informed her the night before on the flight home that he wasn't going to be returning to Medicroy. He didn't want his name associated with them and neither did his family. Dr. Beatrice Clarke, however, was a name that the family was proud to align with and support, and he was more than happy to dive into the frenzy and help her sort through things.

Anthony and Melissa were in Washington making the circuit on the news programs. They effectively deployed the "divide and conquer" technique and were able to appear on all of the major news channels with the help of the paper's PR department. The video that they released shortly after the testimony had gone viral, and the article the next morning was at the top of the news aggregator sites, in addition to pulling up at the top of any Google CBD search.

"#CBDBea – I like that sound of that. I'm dating a hashtag," Jaime teased, handing Bea a cup of coffee.

"Not by choice!" Bea responded adamantly. While the instant flood of positive attention was flattering, it was also overwhelming.

Bea was glad to be at Jaime's for the weekend. His home was like a retreat to her with views that she could lose herself in and surroundings so quiet that she could easily hear the wind rustle the leaves in trees. And then there was Jaime – the man who made her feel like she could accomplish anything while also making her feel like she was the only person in the world.

It was only 8am but it felt like it was noon. The calls and emails had started early, especially for a Saturday. The east coasters had been at it for at least two hours and the west coast was starting to come alive as well. Bea was ignoring the calls for now, letting them go to voicemail to deal with later – until she heard SWEET CAROLINE, BUM BUM BUM sing through her cell phone.

"Mum! I'm so glad it's you!" Bea answered the phone, glad to receive a call from someone she actually knew.

"Lovey, you're all over the place! My phone's been ringing off the hook. Are you OK? Who was that arse that tried to attack you? Tell me he's in jail!" Mary was at the same time both worried for, and immensely proud of, her little girl.

"Yes, Mum. He's in jail. And I'm fine. I'm over at Jaime's and we're sorting through the tons and tons of emails, texts and voicemails that are pouring in. You'll never believe it – Stephen Colbert's show asked me to be a guest on his show! Stephen Colbert!"

"Oh, my! Get a picture with him – and one with Jon Batiste as well! Oh, I'm so happy for you dear! This is all so exciting! And I'm glad that you're at Jaime's. Give Rufus a smooch and a pat on the rear for me."

"Will do. By the way, did you get the CBD I sent you?"

"Yes, love. I got it and I've been taking it every morning and night. I can't tell you how much of a difference it's been making. I'm sleeping like I haven't slept in years and I don't notice the pain as much as I used to. If I really think about it, I can feel it, but other than that, it's barely noticeable at all. And I'm going to start doing Tai Chi with some of the ladies from the Facebook group!"

"Oh, Mum. I'm so glad. And I'm so sorry that I made you wait to try it. I really am. I just didn't know and I was so worried that it would somehow make it worse. Do you forgive me?"

"Of course, dear. Don't give it a second thought. I know you were just looking out for me. Besides, now that you're an expert, you can tell me where to get the good stuff! And I've been thinking, now that I'm moving around more, I'd love to fly out and visit sometime this autumn and see Colorado. It's been so long since I've been able to even think about traveling. I'd love to come for a visit."

"I would love that! Oh, please do!"

"And I can meet the doctor . . ."

"Yes, Mum, you can meet the doctor," Bea laughed, winking at Jaime, who could overhear most of the conversation.

"And I can meet the Mum," Jaime chimed in loudly, so Mary could hear.

"Oh, that would be so lovely!!!!! I'm getting excited just thinking about it!" Mary squealed with joy.

Just then, Rufus jumped up and sprinted to the door, barking wildly. Jaime got up and headed towards the door before the doorbell had even rung.

"Gotta go, Mum. Someone's at the door. Can I call you later?"

"Of course! Have a great day, Beatrice. I'm so proud of you!"

Jaime opened the door to see Adam on the other side of it.

"Hey, come on in," Jaime offered. "Thanks again for flying Bea home. It was a heck of a lot easier to pick her up in Loveland than driving all the way to Denver."

"Happy to do it. Besides, I wanted my dad to meet Bea. And there's the hashtag herself!" Adam teased, as Bea came around the corner to greet him.

"Oh, God. Am I ever going to live this down?"

"Doubt it," replied Adam.

"Not if I have anything to do with it," Jamie chimed in.

Bea, Jaime and Adam spent the next couple hours sorting through the communications that had come through, prioritizing and responding to the glut of invitations and requests that she had received.

Unfortunately, the inevitable happened as well, as Bea was notified that Medicroy Labs was suing her for breach of her non-disclosure agreement. Chad Ellis had given her his contact information on the flight back to Colorado and told her to forward the notification to him immediately. He was confident that it would not hold up in court and had already prepared a draft of a response letter in anticipation of it.

While she knew that she had enormous support from the legal team that was ready to tackle the lawsuit, the experience of actually being notified made her feel incredibly vulnerable and sucked the joy out of all of the positive opportunities coming out of her testimony. Well, that was until "The phone call."

As the morning moved into afternoon and the calls, emails and texts slowed to a dull roar, the trio's adrenaline rush was overridden by their realization that they had not eaten since the day before. Jaime threw some wood into the pizza oven on the patio and showed Adam how to throw pizza dough – quite possibly the ONLY thing that Bea had seen Adam fail miserably at.

Bea searched through Jaime's pantry, cupboards and refrigerator for appetizing and interesting pizza toppings, settling on pickled onions and peppers with a white sauce – a recipe she had been using for years – as well as pepperoni and artichoke with a red sauce. Homemade pizza, fresh from an outdoor pizza oven, was a treat that she was becoming accustomed to since meeting Jaime – a nice perk in a package that included an intelligent, handsome, witty man who loved animals and could make her weak in the knees with just one look, let alone a touch.

The rollercoaster of a day she was experiencing was on a

downswing due to the thought of the lawsuit, coupled with being emotionally drained and hungry. Bea was flustered, and the flurry of contacts from literally hundreds of people left her feeling overwhelmed and unsure of what would be in her best interest to do. She understood that the opportunities coming to her right now would not last forever, though, and doing nothing could be worse than even doing the wrong thing.

She piled the pizza ingredients onto a serving tray and was heading out back when her cell rang and she instinctively answered it.

"Beatrice Clarke, how may I help you?"

"Beatrice, so lovely to reach you. I know how busy you must be, so I'll make this short," the familiar lilting voice replied. "This is Oprah Winfrey and I just wanted to call and congratulate you on your courage - and thank you for standing up and using your voice to call out those who are committing injustices and putting the public at risk. I was forwarded a video of your testimony yesterday and wanted to contact you personally and express my gratitude for your coming forth and exposing your employer's plans to influence politicians into restricting the public's access to CBD. You did an amazing job and I'm so very proud of you."

Bea was in a state of suspended animation. She resembled a figure at Madame Tussaud's Wax Museum – lifelike but frozen solid, her mouth agape and eyes staring straight forward. As hard as she tried, she could not even utter a sound.

"Beatrice? Are you there?" Oprah asked.

"Uh huh," she managed to utter, trying so desperately to regain her composure.

"Are you okay?" Oprah chuckled, obviously experienced in receiving this type of reaction from other calls she had made over the years.

"Yes, ma'am. Yes, ma'am. I'm just so surprised and honored. I mean, this is so unexpected," she finally offered, regaining some control of her brain and bodily functions.

"I'm the one who is honored. I'm doing a series of interviews on up and coming young women who have dared to stand up against powerful forces in politics and I'd like to interview you for the project – if you're interested."

"Yes, ma'am," Bea responded, brain in full gear. "I would love to participate. Thank you for considering me."

"I'll have the producer reach out to you and make the arrangements. I'll let you get back to your afternoon now. We'll be in touch. And, again, congratulations. It took a lot of courage to do what you did."

"Thank you, Miss Winfrey. Thank you so much. Goodbye."

"OH. MY. GOD!!!!!!" she squealed, running out to the back porch, almost tripping over Izzie and dropping the tray in the meantime. "OH MY GOD OH MY GOD OH MY GOD OH

MY GOD!!!!!!!!!" she continued.

"What?" asked Jaime, laughing as he'd never seen Bea in such a state.

"OPRAH WINFREY CALLED ME AND THANKED ME FOR STANDING UP TO MEDICROY AND GELINEX AND WANTS TO INTERVIEW ME!" she yelled at the top of her lungs as Adam grabbed the tray of toppings from her before they ended up spewed all over the patio.

"Oh no, what am I going to wear? I have nothing to wear! I'm going to meet Oprah Winfrey and I have no idea what to wear????" Bea mused, mentally reviewing her wardrobe.

Jaime and Adam looked at each other, impressed with the knee-jerk change in emotion they just witnessed.

Jaime spoke first. "I'm sure that you'll look beautiful no matter what you're wearing," he offered, putting his arms around her to commend her on her big news.

"I'M SO EXCITED!!!!" she screamed, shifting back into hyper mode, nearly bursting Jaime's eardrum.

"How about I start on the pizzas and you do whatever women do when they find out that they're going to be interviewed by Oprah Winfrey – whatever that is," Jaime replied supportively, while backing away to protect himself from any further harm.

"I'm going to take a bubble bath!" Bea decided and ran back

into the house.

Jaime and Adam looked at each other, perplexed and suffering whiplash from the display that they had just been exposed to. They shook their heads and got back to more important things – namely, pizza.

Evening came and the trio relaxed around the fire pit, listening to KBCO Studio C on the Bluetooth speakers that surrounded the patio. They sat there quietly, staring at the flames, recovering from the day of chaos and excitement that they had survived.

NORML had already issued their reply to Medicroy's intent to sue Bea over the NDA, with instructions that all contact was to be directed to them, and that any contact with Bea would be pursued as harassment. Oprah's producer had reached out to Bea while she was taking her bubble bath and emailed her further information shortly after. Adam had secured interviews for Bea on The Late Show with Stephen Colbert, and The Today Show over the following week and was talking with "Meet the Press" about an appearance that Sunday morning.

Jaime stepped away several times to take phone calls and had a discussion with two gentlemen who stopped by in a black Suburban shortly after lunch. They gave him an envelope which he took into his office and placed in a safe under his desk.

Rufus and Izzie spent most of the day lounging in the sun and sniffing each others' butts. Rufus followed Izzie around obediently and wagged his tail when she would occasionally rub up against him and nuzzle him – which wasn't often - but he took what he could get from her. And the frequency was increasing.

All in all, the day was one for the record books – one of the best days of Bea's life. She had no regrets for the choices she'd made and wouldn't change a thing – even if it hadn't resulted in a call from Oprah Winfrey!

Adam headed home for the evening, with the agreement to return in the morning for part two of the aftermath. Jaime doused the fire in the fire pit while Bea gathered up the dishes and brought everything into the kitchen to be cleaned and put away. It had been a magical day and she almost didn't want it to end.

Jaime returned to the house and walked over to the shelves at the far end of the room and picked up a box from the top shelf.

"With all of these interviews coming up, I think I need to get you up to speed on a few things in the industry."

"That would be great. There's just so much information and so many directions to go, I don't even know where to start." Bea walked into the living room and leaned up against the door jamb.

"I thought we could start with a discussion about topicals and the distribution of cb2 receptors on sensory nerve fibers in human skin."

"That would be great. Fill me in. Where do we start?"

"With this," Jaime responded, handing her a box.

Bea opened the box, took out a small bottle and read the label – "Sexual Hemp, CBD lube."

Coming Soon

Purple Haze is the first book in The Cannabinoid Chronicles Series. *Cherry Pie*, the next book in the series, continues Bea's adventures with CDB.

At the end of *Purple Haze*, Bea's new-found fame had generated the hashtag #CBDBea. In *Cherry Pie*, Bea finds being a hashtag isn't all that it's cracked up to be. Fortunately, she has Jaime and Adam to buffer her from the storms that try to knock her down - and the science behind CBD to use as a foundation.

Speaking of Jaime, who IS this guy? There are a lot of unanswered questions surrounding him. Who did Jaime call after Bea received the threatening phone call? What's in the safe under the desk? How does he know the guard at Capitol Hill that helped Derek and Bea sneak out the back after testifying? And who was the guy that knocked Steve Lyons out when he had the needle at Bea's throat?

Bea's life is unfolding in some mysterious and unexpected ways. She will have Merle to contend with and Jaime's sister, Betty, as well.

Fortunately, a little *Cherry Pie* can fix anyone's day.

Author's Note

I hope you enjoyed reading *Purple Haze* and learned a few things in the process about CBD. The purpose of writing this book - and the others in the series - is to reach people, and in an enjoyable way, introduce them to a safe, non-intoxicating cannabinoid that is surrounded in misinformation. If this book piqued your interest, please do some research on CBD and find out how it might impact your life.

Here are some good places to start:
·   **https://www.projectcbd.org/**
·   **http://coscc.org/member-information/** You do not have to be a member to access their research pages. If that page has moved or is not available, go to the main page at http://coscc.org and search from there.
·   And if you REALLY want to go down the rabbit hole, go here: **https://www.ncbi.nlm.nih.gov/pubmed/** Upon the time of this writing, the website has a search bar at the top of the page with a dropdown box to the left of it. Choose PubMed from the dropdown if it's not currently showing. In the search bar, enter "cbd" and whatever symptom or disease you are researching – like "cbd pain" or "cbd seizure dog" (without quotation marks). The most recent publications should populate at the top of the screen. The articles in PubMed are peer reviewed, and therefore the most recent articles are adding to the science or refuting the old science. Older articles may be the original, comprehensive, research. Don't just read one study or article. Keep searching until you find what you need.

To find out about new books, upcoming events and contests, please sign up for my newsletter:
https://cannabinoidchronicles.com
And, of course, my podcast, CBD Talk Podcast. You can find links to all of your favorite streaming platforms here:
https://www.cbdtalkpodcast.com/

Additionally, Harley Damico and Vin Ciffa allowed me to include them in the book. Both are real people and I included their companies in the book as sources of reputable CBD products. You can find their products here:

Homegrown Essentials: **https://ehomegrown.com/**

Clean Green Mart: **https://cleangreenmartbuffalo.com/**

www.ingramcontent.com/pod-product-compliance
Lightning Source LLC
Chambersburg PA
CBHW051449250726
48655CB00001B/322